AIDS IN NEPAL

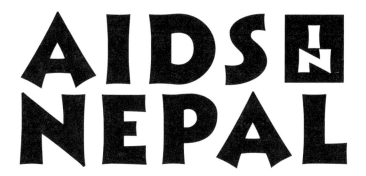

AIDS IN NEPAL

COMMUNITIES CONFRONTING AN EMERGING EPIDEMIC

WRITTEN BY JILL HANNUM

·

Prepared for the American Foundation for AIDS Research
(AmFAR) by the International AIDS Program,
François-Xavier Bagnoud Center for Health and
Human Rights, Harvard School of Public Health

Project Director: Daniel Tarantola, M.D.

AmFAR Published in Association with
SEVEN STORIES PRESS, NEW YORK

American Foundation for AIDS Research (AmFAR)
733 Third Avenue
New York, NY 10017

Published by AmFAR in association with Seven Stories Press,
632 Broadway, New York, NY 10012

Library of Congress Cataloging-in-Publication Data

Hannum, Jill.
    AIDS in Nepal: communities confronting an emerging epidemic /
written by Jill Hannum.
        p. cm.
    ISBN: 1-888363-60-6
    "Prepared for the American Foundation for AIDS Research (AmFAR) by
the International AIDS Program. François-Xavier Bagnoud Center for Health
and Human Rights, Harvard School of Public Health."
    Includes bibliographical references.
        1. AIDS (Disease)—Nepal. I. American Foundation for AIDS Research.
II. François-Xavier Bagnoud Center for Health and Human Rights.
International AIDS Program. III. Title.
RA644.A25H368 1997
362.1'969792'0095496—dc21   97-7915
                                                             CIP

Special discounts are available for classroom use. Please contact AmFAR,
Communications Department: (212) 682-7440.

Cover and book design by Cindy LaBreacht
Front cover photo of Nepali girl by Chris Brown
Back cover photo courtesy of AmFAR Nepal

Printed in the U.S.A.

9 8 7 6 5 4 3 2 1

TABLE OF CONTENTS

HIV incidence and prevalence: Who will care for the sick? / Steep hills, open borders: The disruption of traditional lifestyles / Institutionalized vulnerability: Ethnicity, caste, and social norms / "To be born a daughter is to have an ill fate": The status of women in Nepal / When no one can read the posters: Literacy, HIV, and social development

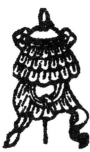Our image of Nepal has long been defined by its mythical representation projected on the screen of our contemporary culture: Nepal is the Shangri-La, a distant Lost Horizon of unconquered mountains and eternal snow, a place where we all aspire to find our spiritual selves.

But for the woman whose husband is returning home from work in a teeming Kathmandu factory, for the aging Nepalese, who, in their own lifetime, have seen their country change from a closed Kingdom to another permeable border in an exploding South East Asian marketplace, Nepal is the people who are daily negotiating with the immediate needs of their everyday lives. Can either of these representations embrace the new reality in Nepal — the haunting specter of the HIV/AIDS pandemic?

Between the dreamscape of the imagination and the enduring rhythms of daily life in the community, there may be a tenuous pathway. It lies somewhere between outdated models of public health and the denial of Nepal's vulnerability to the pandemic of our time in a society seemingly protected by centuries of tradition.

This book is an attempt to scout a new track, one that would be not only sound from a public health perspective but also generated out of the rich cultures of Nepal. It is a trek attended by risk but its destination holds such promise of success, such reduction of human suffering, that it is an exhilarating journey that we are compelled to undertake.

And when we reach the end of that trek, and finally lay our bags down, our eyes will see not only the limitless horizons of mountains in our cultural memory, and not only the microcosm of people struggling with the details of daily lives, but images of our humanity, courageous and dignified, empowered to overcome one of the most severe health crises of our times.

Elizabeth Taylor
Founding National Chairman
American Foundation for AIDS Research

Bel Air, California, 6 April 1996

PREFACE

This book tells the story of an encounter which, at first glance, would have seemed unlikely: it depicts the growing confrontation between the people living in the Himalayan Kingdom of Nepal and the human immunodeficiency virus, HIV.

This unexpected encounter occurred in the early 1990s, in the wake of a global pandemic which had just reached the south Asian subcontinent: once more, HIV had rapidly spread wherever there were waiting opportunities and had found ways to vulnerable populations. In neighboring India, sex workers and their clients in the large and booming metropoles of Bombay and in Madras were trading in unprotected sex; professional blood donors in Bombay were infected by contaminated blood collection equipment; and, in the eastern hilly state of Manipur, drug users had shifted from inhaling opiates to injecting the more powerful heroin, now refined locally.

Given the opportunities, it was merely a question of time for the epidemic to reach Nepal. Economic needs were driving thousands of young girls and women from their impoverished land to the red-light districts of large Indian cities through the complex and thriving networks of the sex trade. Already, some of them had returned to Nepal with symptoms of AIDS. The outcry that attended their homecoming was in itself a sign that the Kingdom was unprepared to face the new realities: Nepal was not immune to AIDS; Nepal was unready to face the coming challenge; Nepal would have a role to play in responding to the new pandemic. No longer just the neighbor's problem, HIV/AIDS had truly become a world pandemic.

In New York, building on a decade of research, the American Foundation for AIDS Research (AmFAR) had reached the same conclusion. AmFAR's interest in Nepal stemmed from a recognition that expanding its mission to the developing world could have multiple benefits: it would enable the HIV/AIDS prevention and research community in the U.S. to share some of its knowledge and resources with an impoverished nation; it would create a tangible example of the universality of the problem it had the mission to address; it would collect knowledge from the developing world's AIDS prevention programs which would enrich its domestic initiatives; and, finally, it would help structure a model to be replicated in other countries. In 1993, after a careful selection of project proposals received from Nepal,

AmFAR began a three-year AIDS community-based prevention program in 17 sites scattered throughout the Kingdom.

The François-Xavier Bagnoud Center for Health and Human Rights of the Harvard School of Public Health had been invited by AmFAR to assist in two ways. First, it was asked to develop an evaluation system for the program. Second, it was expected to build the necessary skills needed locally to ensure that the prevention program would generate new knowledge which, in turn, would guide projects towards the most effective prevention strategies. The Center's research had already led to the development of a framework which expanded the understanding of the HIV/AIDS pandemic. This model stressed the links between individual risk of acquiring HIV infection, risk-taking behaviors and societal factors influencing such behaviors and their safety.

This complex interaction was encompassed in the concept of *vulnerability to HIV/AIDS*, which was a convenient way to express the notion that the societal context within which people are born, raised, initiated to sexuality and are sexually active strongly influences the degree to which an individual is or will be likely to adopt or avoid risk-taking behavior. People may become more vulnerable to HIV/AIDS, for example, as a result of stigmatization and discrimination against them for reason of gender, age, race, sexual orientation, economic status, or cultural, religious, or political affiliation. Indeed, vulnerability to HIV/AIDS is reflected with increased clarity, worldwide, by the focus the pandemic has on individuals, communities and nations who are subjected to marginalization or discrimination. For this reason, any meaningful prevention program would have to address simultaneously the individual factors affecting risk, societal factors influencing this risk, and collective efforts (programs, projects, community mobilization) which, through combined health and social initiatives, would mediate the tensions that exist between individuals and the society of which they are part.

As HIV/AIDS was entering the Kingdom, there were clear signs that the stereotype of "cultural conservatism" often attached summarily to Nepali communities was no more than a veil of vagueness and decency masking the harsh reality of rapidly changing behaviors. In fact, persisting inequality in the status and power of women, growing economic disparity between those who were able to exploit economic opportunities and those who were not, patterns of internal and international mobility induced by the impoverishment of the land or its transfer to a new class of landlords from the cities, had all contributed to a changing order of things. As a consequence, quests for employment and means of survival had set the stage for sexual behaviors to change, for sexually transmitted diseases to spread and for HIV to set in.

The immediate objective of the AmFAR initiated program in Nepal was to enable people to protect themselves and their sexual partners against HIV/AIDS through information, education and access to means of prevention. The program also aimed to reduce people's individual and collective vulnerability to HIV/AIDS through the creation and enhancement of skills needed for alternate income generation, such as literacy. More importantly, the development of field projects would yield a better understanding of the societal factors that place some people at a higher risk than others in acquiring HIV and other sexually-transmitted diseases in specific community settings.

In Nepal, there are many health problems that compete with HIV in terms of the morbidity and mortality burden they place on the population. But because of the unique clarity with which HIV illuminates societal factors influencing health, it provides an effective entry-point to reveal the deeply rooted societal causes of risk-taking behaviors which, consequently, lead to illness and premature death. A clearer vision of HIV/AIDS will help uncover the determinants of our physical, mental and social well-being, thereby allowing us to take a more direct responsibility for our own lives.

This book includes chapters written by Jill Hannum, boxes contributed by other authors and a substantial list of references to community-focused initiatives that have been carried out since 1990—a date which coincides with the emergence of a large number of non-governmental organizations in Nepal. Also appended is a list of recommended readings for those either in or outside Nepal who wish to learn more about the body of experience and knowledge accumulated through health, anthropological and social research in this country.

In gathering the stories that constitute this book, Jill Hannum has listened, with her ears and her heart, to the testimony of people who are at the forefront of the response to HIV/AIDS in Nepal. She has transcribed very skillfully and vividly the lessons learned by non-governmental and governmental organizations during their two years of hard work. She tells the story of the community-based organizations, which as it unfolds, reveals the many discoveries that they made through their interaction with young people and adults—some educated and economically secure, others poor and illiterate—across the country. She has offered these stories trusting that the voices of the people she met in the Himalayan Kingdom will be stopped neither by mountain ranges nor indifference but will be echoed and carried over distance and time in an unyielding message of hope.

Daniel Tarantola, M.D.
Director of the International AIDS Program,
François-Xavier Bagnoud Center for Health and
Human Rights, Harvard School of Public Health

Boston, Massachusetts, 23 January 1997

ACKNOWLEDGMENTS

AmFAR's community-based HIV/AIDS prevention efforts in Nepal were the result of close international collaboration between a large number of participants from within and outside Nepal. The program was initially designed by Rev. Margaret R. Reinfeld, former Director of the AmFAR HIV/AIDS Education and Prevention Program, with the assistance of Vivia Dennis, David S. Hausner, Molly Lucas and, from beginning to end, Mary McMechan, Project Supervisor. It was implemented by seventeen non-governmental organizations listed in Appendix B of this book.

AmFAR wishes to extend its heartfelt thanks to His Majesty's Government of the Kingdom of Nepal without whose help the project could not have been realized. We are indebted to those Nepali officials whose interest and commitment were also extremely helpful: Jagadishwar Upadhyay, Ministry of Health; Govind Adhikari and Krishna Prasad Khanal, Social Welfare Council; Bapal Gopal Vaidya, National Planning Commission; and Hemang Dixit, Institute of Medicine. Finally, special thanks are extended to B.B. Karki who played a key role in mobilizing a national response to HIV/AIDS in Nepal.

The voices of many Nepali NGO leaders and staff are heard throughout this book: Gopi Raj Adhikari (WICOM), Meera Ariyal

(ABC Nepal), Rajendra Bhadra (B.P. Memorial), Gita Bhatta (LALS), Govin Bhatta (CRDS), Bal Ram Dahal (WICOM), Joyoty Kumar Roy Danuwar (DSS), Shamby Dhital (LALS), Verona Dixit (CDS), Gita Ghatta (LALS), Rita Gurung (WICOM), Rajendra Gurung (WICOM), Lava Joshi (B.P. Memorial), R.P. Kandel (ICH), Hira Gharti Magar (SAFE), Shiba Hari Maharjan (LALS), Bhagawati Nepal (MANK), Ashok Nepali (SAFE), Kamal Nepali (SAFE), Raj Kumar Nepali (SAFE), Barav Phatak (WICOM), Chet Raj Pant (ICH), Dilip Pariyar (SAFE), Shambu Phital (LALS), Jalpa Pradhan (ABC Nepal), Soma Rai (NESCORD), Binayak Rajbhandari (WOREC), Sujata Rana (LALS), Azeliya Ranjitkar, Navaraj Raj Raut (WOREC), D.R. Sharma (WICOM), Sharad Sharma (CDS), Lal Singh Tamang (WICOM), and Pradeepta Upadhyay (WICOM). We are grateful to the above individuals and to others who, throughout Nepal, so graciously granted interviews which provided the substance of this book.

We wish to congratulate and thank other NGO leaders and staff persons, including AmFAR staff members, who carried out or provided support to the program with great dedication: Savita Acharya (NAPCP), Kamala Adhikari (WOREC), Bruce Anderson (AmFAR), Jagya Raj Bhatta (ICH), Lek Raj Bhatta (SC/US), Pushpa Basnet (SCF/UK), Nahalkul K. C. (BASE), Mariann Caprino (AmFAR), Eleanor Cicerchi (AmFAR), Dilli Bahadur Chaudhary (BASE), Chandra Bdr. Choudhary (BASE), Hem Raj Kumar Danwar (DSS), Gochi Denar (CHDC), Ashok Bikram Deo (NNSWA), R.R. Dhungana (ICH), Geeta Ghimire (AmFAR/Nepal), Purnima Gurung (CHDC), L.N. Gyawali (CRDS), Kashi R. Gyawali (CRDS), Ivo Heast (SCF/UK), Moti Ingnam (NESCORD), Ernie Jackson (AmFAR), Ashok Bikhran Jairu (NNSWA), Shanta Kafle (WATCH), Shanta Karki (WATCH), Ashesh Malla (WICOM),

Sabitri Malla (WICOM), Sundar Mulepati (SC/US), Jagi Devi Ode (NNSWA), Ashok Pandey (NNSWA), R.P. Panthi (CRDS), Dilip Pariyar (SAFE), Aaron Peak (LALS), Laxmi Pokhrel (CHDC), Meena Poudel (WATCH), Navin Pyakuryal (SC/US), Renu Rajbhandari (WOREC), Arun K. Rai (NESCORD), Chanda Rai (SC/US), Geeta Ravi (AmFAR/Nepal), Mohammad Shamsuddin (SC/US), Sharad Sharma (CDS), Amina Shresta (NCWCA), Anju Shresta (NCWCA), Ganesh Shresta (AmFAR/Nepal), Laxmi P. Shresta (CDS), Rheka Shresta (AmFAR/Nepal), Soni Shresta (SCF/UK), Arjun Sigdel (WICOM), Manisha Singh (LALS), Amina Shresta (NCWCA), Hari Maya Subba (SC/US), Naveen Suba (AmFAR), Ravi Thapa (AmFAR/Nepal), B.P. Upadhaya (NAPCP), Aruna Uprety (WOREC), Renu Wagle (NCWCA), and Gary Paul Wright (AmFAR).

Technical support was provided to the Nepal program by Sara Back, Pushpa Baht, Steve Bezruchka, Becky Bunnell, Manuel Carballo, R.R. Dhungana, Matthew Frey, Ganesh Gurung, Subhash Hira, Paul Janssen, Keith Leslie, Gheeta Sodhi and Sundar Sundararaman. All of these professionals contributed their time, competence and energy—and several of them their voices—to this monograph. We appreciate very much their contributions.

Many of the photographs contained in this book represent the outstanding work of Christopher Brown. Chris Brown traveled extensively with us, generously donating his time to meet the people of Nepal and to so artfully record the ongoing work there. His contribution enriched this book tremendously.

We extend our warmest thanks to William Fisher and Ganesh Gurung, who helped keep this project on track and reviewed early versions of this document from an anthropological perspective. With the help of research assistants at the Harvard School of Public Health, they helped build an extensive bibliography on community-based health and social programs in Nepal (Annex 1)—a resource which should aid all those committed to improving the welfare of the Nepali people. We also wish to acknowledge Thomas Cox, Teguest Guerma, Jonathan Mann and Masumi Watase for their insight and cooperation. Finally, thanks to Elizabeth Marlin, of AmFAR, for her proofreading and editing support.

This project would have never happened without the vision and commitment of the AmFAR Board of Directors. In particular, we acknowledge Mathilde Krim, Mervyn Silverman and Elizabeth Taylor who, in a true spirit of international solidarity, inspired this collaborative response to HIV/AIDS so far away from American shores. We also especially thank Jerome J. Radwin, CEO, for his wise counsel and personal support.

We warmly thank the funders of AmFAR's International Program who provided the financial resources needed to implement this project. We are particularly endebted to Hiro Yamagata for his outstanding personal generosity. We are also extremely grateful to Marella Agnelli for her extraordinary efforts in connection with "Art Against AIDS Venice"; to Sao Schlumberger for her critical role in "Cinema Against AIDS" (Cannes); to Richard Marshall, Junji Ito, Nam June Paik, Robert Rauschenberg, and Hiroshi Teshigahara for their time, generosity and expertise with regard to "Art Against AIDS Japan," and to all those individuals whose generosity made these efforts such a success. Finally, we would like to thank Anne Livet for her fundraising expertise, the staff of Savvy Management for their advice regarding public relations, and Delphine Farber, of AmFAR, for her tireless energy and skills in coordinating international events. We hope they are proud of the work they enabled AmFAR to accomplish.

The evaluation of this project and the production of this book were undertaken on behalf of AmFAR by the François-Xavier Bagnoud Center for Health and Human Rights of the Harvard School of Public Health. The Center was founded with a grant made possible by Albina du Boisrouvray. We are indebted to her for her commitment to public health and human rights.

The publication of this book was made possible by Seven Stories Press. Dan Simon and Jon Gilbert at Seven Stories took on this unconventional project, gave generously of their time and expertise, and provided their uncompromising commitment throughout. In addition, we especially want to thank Cindy LaBreacht for her beautiful design and layout and for executing her work in record time; she truly made this project come to life.

Most importantly, we are profoundly grateful to Jill Hannum who, with great modesty and talent, so effectively gave a voice to those seldom heard on the international scene: The women, men and children of Nepal.

Paul Corser, Program Officer
American Foundation for AIDS Research
New York, NY, USA

Sally Morrison, V.P. External Affairs
American Foundation for AIDS Research
New York, NY, USA

Daniel Tarantola, Director, International AIDS Program
François-Xavier Bagnoud Center for Health and
Human Rights, Harvard School of Public Health,
Boston, MA, USA

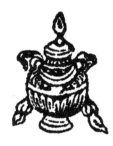

In March 1995, I agreed to take an assignment to document the "lessons learned" by 16 Nepali NGOs doing HIV/AIDS prevention and education. The NGOs were midway through a three year grant cycle, and the funder, the American Foundation for AIDS Research, felt it would be valuable to write up their experiences. It was decided that I would attend a week-long skills development workshop for the NGOs in Kathmandu, then go into the field for in-depth interviews. I was also to talk to the AmFAR technical assistance staff, go through files, surveys and reports, and meet with representatives of WHO and the National

AIDS Program before going home to write what eventually became this book. I thought it sounded doable.

I have been a free-lance writer and editor for over 20 years, often focusing on issues relating to HIV/AIDS. I thought I was well prepared to work in Nepal—I live in the rural mountains without many amenities and I've traveled widely. That helped, but Nepal proved to be unique unto itself. The planned two week stay stretched into a month, and I later decided a year might have been adequate. Nepal and deadlines do not mix. Everything was much more complex than expected and took longer. This was especially true of conducting interviews through an interpreter. Perhaps two thirds of the people I interviewed spoke English, some fluently. At the other end of the spectrum were Tharu villagers who spoke no English and little Nepali. My warmest thanks go to AmFAR Program Manager Azeliya Ranjitkar who accompanied me on site visits, arranged interviews, translated, and filled in necessary background information. Her kindness and good humor were unfailing—traits I found common in Nepal.

My first week in Kathmandu gave me a chance to watch the NGOs interact among themselves and with the technical assistance staff and to listen to their prepared presentations. Over the next three weeks I spoke to representatives from 11 NGOs, some rather briefly, others over the course of two or three days. I went to factories in Kathmandu and Pokhara and to villages near Nepalgung and Pokhara. I walked through Kathmandu with needle-exchange outreach workers, spent a day with Badi commercial sex workers and sat at an HIV/AIDS information booth on the Indian border in 114 degree heat. My aim was to get the voices not only of NGO directors, but of their field staff and target populations as well—voices not often heard, and certainly unused to being listened to.

But it is the NGOs' voices, not the individual voices, that are the focus of this study. The quotations attributed to NGOs in this book are amalgams of several interviews and are designed to tell the story of whatever lesson is being illustrated. I have tried to use the speakers' phrasing when possible in order to preserve the character of the exchange, but to say that the narratives have been condensed would be the broadest of understatements. Quotations attributed by name to individuals are theirs alone, though they may have been translated or made more concise.

It was not my assignment to evaluate the NGOs' performance or their program's impact but to document their efforts and achievements. The scientific evaluation is a task for professional evaluators down the line. What is valuable at this stage is an ethnographic study, to hear people tell in their own words how they increased their capacity to identify and resolve the problems they faced.

The chapters that focus on specific target groups are intended to mimic the NGOs' process of gathering and analyzing data for research and drawing conclusions or hypotheses. They begin with a problem statement, define the targeted population and why it is at risk for HIV infection, then present data gathered through the interviews. Ideally, this format makes a logical progression. To conclude each chapter, I have drawn together a few points about the main issues affecting the population in focus and what interventions for them may need to be investigated in the future.

Long after my return, the people whose lives I touched, however briefly, are still with me every day. I remember a tiny woman at a construction site who stood patiently while the basket on her back was loaded with what seemed like 100 bricks, then walked away with a slow grace that seemed impossible. I remember that I met, indeed, saw, very few people older than I am. I remember urging an obviously unwell NGO field worker to stop shepherding me around and take the afternoon off. "Why do you care?" he asked. It wasn't a hostile comment; he was genuinely surprised that I would be concerned for his welfare.

HIV has the potential to devastate Nepal, and there seems to be very little standing in its way. Yet the NGOs have managed to do so much in so short a time with so little that it would be beyond the comprehension of even a modestly-funded organization in the U.S.—no mail, no telephone, no vehicles, no infrastructure. And, for many, there is also a deep knowledge that there is no one they can rely on consistently but themselves and their community. In the long run, that knowledge may be a source of strength, but for now, they need and deserve all the help they can get.

Jill Hannum

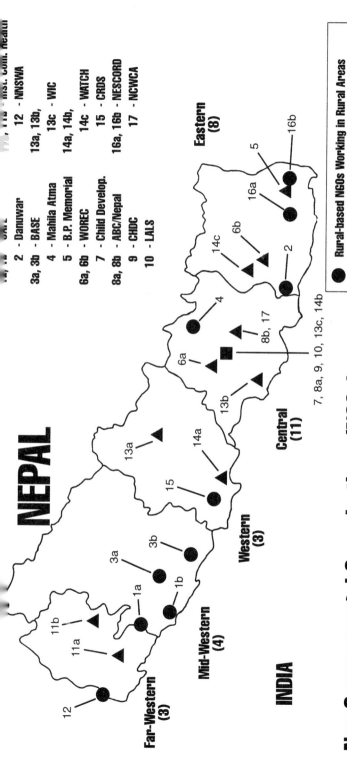

Non-Governmental Organizations (NGOs)
Locations and Project Sites

NEPAL

Far-Western (3)
Mid-Western (4)
Western (3)
Central (11)
Eastern (8)

INDIA

Legend:
- ● Rural-based NGOs Working in Rural Areas
- ▲ Kathmandu-based NGOs Working in Rural Areas
- ■ Kathmandu-based NGOs Working in Kathmandu

2 - Danuwar
3a, 3b - BASE
4 - Mahila Atma
5 - B.P. Memorial
6a, 6b - WOREC
7 - Child Develop.
8a, 8b - ABC/Nepal
9 - CHDC
10 - LALS
12 - NNSWA
13c - WIC
14c - WATCH
15 - CRDS
16a, 16b - NESCORD
17 - NCWCA

"1986 was when Nepal began to think it really needed to intervene in the HIV/AIDS question. That was before there were any HIV cases here, but the population throughout the country was already vulnerable. Yet for the next six or seven years, the activities hardly went outside the Kathmandu valley. That's a pity, because once we realized it could sweep the country, activities should have been started everywhere. We don't know how bad the situation is, but we can conclude from certain indications that somehow God has been saving Nepal from the worst catastrophe."

—DR. B.B. KARKI, FORMER DIRECTOR, NATIONAL AIDS PROGRAM

CHAPTER 1

AN INVISIBLE EPIDEMIC: HIV/AIDS IN THE CONTEXT OF NEPAL

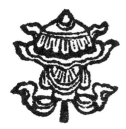 HIV/AIDS is a nearly invisible epidemic in Nepal, the world's tenth poorest country. It arrived relatively recently and has developed and spread almost without notice. A surprisingly large percentage of Nepal's 20 million people have never heard of the epidemic, and among those who have, fear, superstition and misinformation about HIV/AIDS abound. People fear catching it from a sneeze or a bus seat. Families have banished members suspected of being HIV positive. The crucial question today is how quickly the recently energized movement to foster HIV awareness and education can take root in this low incidence country and begin to slow the spread of the virus.

After a long period of denial, the government of Nepal established a National AIDS Program in 1986 with support from the World Health Organization and joined later by other international donors. Soon, a growing number of indigenous Non-Governmental Organizations (NGOs) began prevention and awareness activities, often with support from international NGOs (INGOs). In 1993, the American Foundation for AIDS Research (AmFAR) began providing funds and logistical support for 17 Nepali NGOs to bring HIV/AIDS awareness and prevention information to a broad spectrum of communities throughout the country. Each NGO developed its own objectives, strategies and work plan, and every project was combined with an AmFAR research component to learn what factors affect a community's vulnerability to HIV and how that knowledge can be used to improve prevention programs.

The AmFAR partner NGOs are working with and in their communities to develop appropriate and effective responses to the threat of HIV. Often, this means integrating HIV/AIDS messages into a much broader strategy of community development that also provides such things as loans to buy pigs, literacy classes in factories, or education for sex workers' children. Many of these NGOs have faced opposition to their programs, stigmatization of their target populations and discrimination against their staff, as well as the considerable challenge of working in one of world's least developed countries.

The constellation of factors contributing to the difficulty of controlling the spread of HIV in Nepal is outlined in this chapter. Some of the elements are almost unique to Nepal. Others are common to many poor countries. But what truly links Nepal with the rest of the world is the fact that there, as everywhere, marginalization of and discrimination against certain communities is linked with their vulnerability to HIV infection.

HIV INCIDENCE AND PREVALENCE: WHO WILL CARE FOR THE SICK?

"Nepal is a low prevalence country. But there are a lot of potential risks. HIV is low still, even among the high risk groups. But STDs are high among these risk groups and STD rates can give a direct idea of HIV risk. The epicenter of the epidemic is Kathmandu, but even where HIV is still not introduced, that day it is introduced, it will spread very quickly, because STD prevalence is so high. It is the time now to do prevention. Tomorrow it will be too late." —*Dr. Teguest Guerma, Medical Officer, WHO Global Program on AIDS, Kathmandu*

Even at this early stage of the epidemic, Nepal's formal health care system is ill equipped to respond. The first AIDS case was diagnosed in 1988. As of October 1995, 173 males and 158 females had been diagnosed with HIV. Of those 331 cases, 49 had AIDS. However, current reporting is likely to seriously underestimate the number of cases. This is because HIV/AIDS public awareness is low, access to medical care and/or testing facilities is extremely limited, and stigmatization mitigates against knowing one's status. The actual number of HIV infections is estimated to be between 5,000 and 7,000. In its best-case scenario, the World Health Organization predicts 100,000 HIV infections in Nepal by 2000, in the worst case, 300,000.

In 1992, Nepal had 12,352 doctors (outside the Kathmandu valley, one for every 53,000 people) and 4,848 hospital beds.

Especially in rural Nepal (where 90% of the population lives), only a very small fraction of the population will see a doctor if they are ill, though a greater number will visit traditional healers, pharmacists or medics. The formal health system is structurally weak, lacks resources and already struggles with a broad spectrum of health problems in a country where the average life expectancy is only 53 years. Even in its early stages, HIV infection increases vulnerability to TB, other respiratory infections and diarrhea, three of Nepal's most severe health problems. (Others include malaria, malnutrition, meningitis, leprosy and STDs). Nepal devotes 5 percent of its national budget to health, but spends less than half the per capita average of other poor countries.

The mode of HIV transmission in Nepal is almost exclusively from man to woman and woman to man. Commercial sex workers (134), their clients (164) and housewives (16) account for almost all cases. Nine injecting drug users have been diagnosed with HIV, but the mode of transmission is listed as sexual. Blood transfusion and perinatal transmission account for one case each. As in other countries, the great majority of HIV infections are among young people.

STEEP HILLS, OPEN BORDERS:
THE DISRUPTION OF TRADITIONAL LIFESTYLES

In Nepal, the land itself plays a role both in increasing people's vulnerability to HIV and the complexity of implementing prevention activities. The Himalayas cover the northern third of the country from east to west, bordering China. To their south lies a long east-west stretch of lower mountains whose southern flanks flatten into the Terai, a fertile, sub-tropical plain spanning the border with India. These contours have played a major role in helping to determine the geographical and social diversity that characterizes Nepal. They can also make economic development and access to services such as health care and education extremely difficult for some communities.

Compounding the problem is the fact that Nepal has no rail system and the highway system, though developing, is still limited. The road system is best developed in the Terai and the Kathmandu Valley and many of the roads under construction are designed to link villages to urban areas, thus facilitating migration and urbanization. Most goods and people, however, still move by foot and animal, and distance is often measured in walking days. One NGO budgets funds for porters so a generator and equipment to show their AIDS awareness video can be carried to otherwise inaccessible sites.

In Nepal, the topography, environmental degradation, poverty and economic migration are all linked, and they combine to increase vulnerability to HIV. The 90 percent of the population that is rural has traditionally worked small agricultural plots, created local crafts and/or been hired out locally for wages. But a combination of forces has been undermining rural self-sufficiency. Most of this population has little or no cash income and lives in absolute poverty. Nepal is one of the most densely populated mountainous countries in the world, and the population is growing by 2.1 percent per year. From the perspective of the land's ability to support a population, all of Nepal can be considered heavily populated. In the hills and mountains, where families are more likely to own or control their own fields, the land is marginal for agriculture and unforgiving of environmental insult. In more fertile areas, particularly the Terai, much of the land is controlled by relatively few landlords. Though not legally sanctioned, a feudal-style system still persists in certain areas and it allows owners to exploit labor and restrict or deny traditional access.

Population growth and limited access to additional arable land have had and continue to have a devastating effect on Nepal's environment. People are forced to expand available farmland into forests and onto steep slopes, and the demand for firewood has become extremely high. Once heavily forested, only 27 percent of Nepal's original tree cover remains, though 60 percent is considered necessary to maintain environmental balance. The effect of the yearly monsoon rains on the deforested and eroded slopes can be catastrophic. Finally, in addition to the economic pressure caused by growing environmental degradation, many of Nepal's people are facing growing competition posed by lower-priced imports of the same products made in their home industries.

In response to these economic burdens, increasing numbers of villagers (predominantly men but often women and sometimes whole families) are migrating in search of work. In some areas, growing numbers of women and girls choose or are trafficked into full or part-time sex work to generate income. Many Nepalis seeking paid work turn toward India, with which Nepal maintains an open border and where a major AIDS epidemic has developed over the past six years. Some 800,000 migrant laborers and thousands of Nepali transportation workers regularly cross into India and back, and an estimated 100,000 to 200,000 Nepali girls and women are reported to be working in the sex industry in India.

INSTITUTIONALIZED VULNERABILITY: ETHNICITY, CASTE, AND SOCIAL NORMS

Cultural, social and religious factors in Nepal can increase vulnerability to HIV for some populations and can also make it difficult for NGOs to implement prevention programs and get them accepted. According to figures from the government of Nepal, the country's population is 90 percent Hindu, 5.3 percent Buddhist and 2.7 percent Muslim. However, these figures are widely disputed within Nepal where Buddhist and Hindu practices can be uniquely and inextricably intertwined and often mingle with local animist practices as well. In general, Nepal's social and political leaders tend to reflect the orthodox beliefs of the "higher" Hindu castes: men's and women's roles follow narrowly defined scripts, there is very little room for individualism or iconoclasm, and religious and family duties are of paramount importance. These are the values that seem to have shaped Nepal's public self-image as that of a country where women are virgins until marriage, spouses are monogamous, and homosexuality does not exist. That this is not born out in everyday life is rarely publicly acknowledged. Indeed, it is uncommon for anyone to admit that there is such a discrepancy. Some AmFAR partner NGOs have been surprised to find that careful investigation in the field has changed their understanding of what is and is not possible and acceptable in Nepal's societies. One NGO, for example, was told that because of student shyness it is "not possible" to teach sexuality in school programs. Their experience, however, has encouraged them to believe that such a crucial HIV/AIDS prevention tool could indeed be introduced in Nepal, though it would require an innovative curriculum stressing peer educators and student participation.

Nepali NGO workers often characterize their country as one of the least open places in the world with respect to sex and sexuality. While not universally true (among some populations, the matter is quite open) many people, especially women, do exhibit a shyness or reticence about discussing sexual matters, and the NGOs have had to struggle to learn to circumvent it. For example, when a physician from one AmFAR NGO asked to examine a village man at an STD clinic, the man is reported to have replied: "Sir, I have three wives and none of them has ever seen my organ. Why should I show it to you?" Nepali men and women generally do not touch in public or discuss sexual matters in front of the opposite sex, especially if related by blood or marriage, and NGOs report that accurate information on the topic is wholly unavailable to most of the population.

Given the broad diversity of Nepal's castes and ethnicities, it is difficult and often unwise to generalize about the population, despite the apparent uniformity of its public image. Nepal has at least 75 ethnic groups and some 50 languages, almost all of which are Indo-Aryan, Tibeto-Burman, or some mixture of the two. Broadly put, the closer a group is to the Indo-Aryan end of the scale, the more likely it is to espouse adherence to the caste system, arranged child-marriage, and minimal participation of women in education and employment. Tibeto-Burman groups are more likely to be relatively egalitarian with respect to both gender and caste.

In Nepal, caste and ethnicity determine one's place in a society that is structured on the basis of "Jot." This can be translated as "type," and the term encompasses the complex and intertwined area of defining characteristics such as caste and ethnicity. Brahmins, Chhetris and Thakuris are at the top of Nepal's caste hierarchy and hold most positions of power in Nepali society. The social elite have what might be described as a Brahminized life style, and it is widely emulated by the upwardly mobile from other groups who adopt some orthodox Brahmin ways, such as earlier marriages for their daughters. At the other end of the spectrum are the exploited and discriminated against Tamang and Tharu communities and Nepal's several million "untouchables" (the actual figure is widely disputed) including the Badi and Danuwar people.

Although discrimination based on caste was legally abolished in 1963, the traditional hierarchies still exert a powerful influence on social organization and status. This has the effect of the institutionalization of poverty, exploitation of labor, lack of access to social services, abuse of human rights, and low status for females. The Danuwar director of an AmFAR NGO asserts that "Real Nepal is the ethnic groups of Nepal, and institutionalized discrimination makes them vulnerable." His use of the term ethnic group is clearly meant to distinguish Tibeto-Burman groups such as the Danuwar, Tamang and Tharu from the Hindu caste groups.

"TO BE BORN A DAUGHTER IS TO HAVE AN ILL FATE" (NEPALI PROVERB): THE STATUS OF WOMEN IN NEPAL

"A village woman I know of is typical. She has two children and works from dawn to dusk at home and in the fields. The adult males in her family—father-in-law, two brothers-in-law, husband—make leather goods to sell. They make a good income, but she owns only one sari and one blouse. So, even if this family is not poor, the woman is poor."—*Azeliya Ranjitkar, AmFAR Program Manager*

For half the population of Nepal, all the factors that increase HIV risk and vulnerability are compounded by having been born female. Whatever a woman's caste, class, ethnicity, or economic status, she will always have lower status than men. Sons play a key role in Hindu religion and culture, and Nepal may have the highest preference for boy children in the world. Girls traditionally have less access to good nutrition, health care or education, despite the fact that their contribution to the household's economy is often far greater than boys'. This early neglect, combined with high fertility rates and lack of medical care during pregnancy and birth, makes women's life expectancy lower than men's.

Females are dependent first on their fathers, then on their husbands. Marriage is almost universal and the bride is usually in her teens (sometimes as young as 13). Modern law and some customs permit divorce, but, like remarriage, it is accepted in some communities but quite uncommon in others. Widowhood, for example, can create tremendous hardship for high-caste Hindu women, but is less of a burden in those communities where women can earn and keep their own income. The lives of higher caste women are often the most restricted, and although untouchable women are the most exploited in society, they have more equality within their caste. Gender inequality makes it especially difficult for women to negotiate safer sex with their husbands or know their sexual histories. A woman who refuses to have sex with her husband risks divorce or having him take a second wife. Having two—or sometimes three—wives is widely accepted in Nepal and may be practiced by men who can afford the additional economic responsibility. In a few communities, women may have more than one husband.

Women play a key role in Nepal's labor force, mainly in agriculture, cottage industry and factory work, but they are invariably paid less than men. Lacking education and marketable skills, many women turn to commercial sex work as a response to economic pressures. In some areas of Nepal young women may be sold into the sex trade by parents, relatives or brokers—often at an early age. Ironically, such devaluation of females and their treatment as commodities is countered by a widespread cultural veneration of motherhood, the worship of female deities, and, often, a strong, participatory role for fathers in the care of their children.

The role of women in Nepal is slowly changing. The constitution grants them equality and the vote, and by law 5 percent of all political candidates must be women. Women can be found in small numbers in many professions, and *Yosha*, the country's first periodical devoted to women's issues, recently began publication. Women play a prominent role in several AmFAR partner NGOs, particularly those that focus on creating social, economic and legal awareness among women and girls. Such positions of relative privilege are available to only a tiny fraction of Nepal's women, however. For the vast majority, it remains true that it is an ill fate to be born a daughter.

WHEN NO ONE CAN READ THE POSTERS: LITERACY, HIV, AND SOCIAL DEVELOPMENT

Many of the factors already discussed—physical and cultural isolation, gender inequality, poverty and migration—can combine to limit people's access to information and education, both key components in the struggle against HIV/AIDS. Widespread illiteracy compounds this problem. Government schools are free through the fourth grade, but many rural areas still have no government elementary schools, and those that do often lack qualified teachers and supplies. The situation is further complicated by the fact that many rural people speak little or no Nepali. A common estimate is that 25 percent of men and 12 percent of women are literate, but statistics vary widely, and people with only limited skills may be counted. Literacy is lowest in rural areas where, even for those who can read, access to print materials is limited. Other sources of information are radio, which reaches over two thirds of the population, and television, to which most urban dwellers have some access. (Nepal has one TV station and can receive radio and television from India.)

The AmFAR partner NGOs have found that the more education people have, the easier it is for them to understand messages not only about HIV/AIDS but also about matters of general health and welfare that could make a crucial difference in their lives. So, while they are busy designing creative informational materials for people who cannot read, many NGOs are also offering literacy programs. As one NGO emphasizes, "Comprehensive literacy empowers communities for development," and integrating HIV prevention into the context of Nepal's greater needs may be key to its success.

NEPAL'S RESPONSE TO AIDS

Nepal's National AIDS Program (NAP) was implemented in 1986. Government decision makers were slow to respond, partly because of lack of resources, but also because, as in many other countries, AIDS was dismissed as a problem of foreigners or of stigmatized populations such as sex workers and injecting drug users. This attitude has changed within the past two years and the government has committed itself to funding and implementing a national AIDS policy.

Unfortunately, the funding is extremely limited. A 1994 World Bank report estimated that 84 percent of the HIV/AIDS-related expenditures in Nepal in FY 1995 would come from foreign donors, but government sources were anticipated to contribute $282,240 U.S. It is extremely unlikely that that goal was even approached. NAP's current yearly budget, for example, is estimated at only about $5,000 U.S.—though NAP does not represent all the government's HIV/AIDS expenditures.

Early on, the NAP focused on case detection and tracking. Recent focus is more on developing national information/education /communication (IEC) activities and strategy. It is also working with The World Health Organization, the European Economic Community, the United Nations and the U.S. Agency for International Development to develop targeted STD/HIV prevention programs in selected districts. Additional NAP responsibilities include surveillance and training health personnel. Given its other priorities, the NAP has had few resources to devote to strategic planning, policy development or technical support for NGOs, and few activities have been developed in the area of care for HIV and AIDS patients. NAP also suffers because the leadership staff is politically appointed and subject to sudden reassignment.

THE STIGMA OF A SEXUALLY TRANSMITTED DISEASE

Any organization seeking to target HIV positive individuals in Nepal has a particularly difficult task. Few people know their HIV status and few who know they are positive are willing to come forward. Stigmatization can be thorough and brutal. In the past, photos, names and addresses of people with HIV were publicized. This has changed, but there are still strong incentives to hide one's health status. But negative attitudes can be changed. One NGO, which is working with HIV positive women who are returning to live with their families, has found that there are few problems with acceptance if the organization talks with the woman's family and organizes meetings with the community to answer questions and provide education. When I asked people to tell me their experience with community attitudes toward people known to or believed to have HIV or STDs, I found encouraging evidence of acceptance and sympathy as well as the expected fear and rejection.

"STDs are considered a bad disease in our society because they are associated with illegal sex. We have an extended family system, but people with STDs get pushed away. I interviewed a woman who came back from Bombay with HIV. Her family accepted her because no one knew why she was sick. But when she went to the hospital in Kathmandu, it was rumored she had AIDS. Then an NGO pressured her to get tested. After her family learned she was positive, they made her stay alone in a shed and threw her food to her. She

had a little business selling liquor, and people did buy, even though they knew she had HIV. They felt sorry for her. So the village treated her better than her family. Then WOREC took her in and gave her counseling and training. She slowly got back with her family and had some savings from income generation projects to put a down payment on a little hotel. I expected a lot of negative feedback to my article on her, but there was none. Now, people say she won't live long."
—*Azeliya Ranjitkar, AmFAR Program Manager*

"A man in Jhapa talked openly to a peer educator about his STD symptoms and people overheard. Word got around. Then his mother-in-law died. Now, in Nepal, everyone helps out the family at the time of a death, that is a very strong tradition. This man needed to borrow a bike to go into the jungle for materials to weave a mat to wrap her body in. This is also a tradition. But because he 'had an STD,' he was refused the loan, because people thought they could catch something from the bicycle seat if he used it. It took the peer educator four weeks to convince people that wasn't so."—*B.P. Memorial Health Foundation*

"There was a fellow from nearby who came back from Bombay. He was very weak and he was embarrassed to sit with us. When we asked about his health, he just said, 'This is my disease.' He used to be very outspoken and his behavior changed so much, we suspected he had AIDS. He may have known, but he didn't tell us. We knew about AIDS from radio and TV, and some of us had little pocket calendars from family planning with information about HIV on it. We knew enough not to be afraid we would catch it from him. I don't know how bad his death was, but it is hard to see someone 30 or 35 die. It is not good to die so young. So we are afraid of AIDS."—*Kalidas Lamachine, farmer, Bagmara*

FROM DEFORESTATION TO PROSTITUTION

The World Development Report 1996 showed Nepal, with a per capita income of $200 U.S., to be the tenth poorest country in the world. It must also be remembered that this represents an average income, which is inflated by a small number of relatively wealthy people living in the urban areas. In fact, 87 percent of the Nepali population live in rural areas with an annual income that is far less than $200 U.S. Many of these people survive in absolute poverty and are deprived of even basic needs. This poverty is further accelerated by a population increase of 2.5 percent each year which makes Nepal, with 148 people per square kilometer in 1996, the most densely populated among the mountainous countries.

Poverty has driven people to encroach upon the forests, expand their farmlands on to the hard and unforgiving slopes and, sometimes, to cut down trees recklessly to ensure their very survival. As a result, between 1961 and 1971, Nepal lost 50 percent of its forest cover. With the overall destruction of 4.5 million hectares of national forest, the total forested area in Nepal has been reduced to about 1 million hectares—only about 27 percent of the total area of the country. Meanwhile, it has been estimated that in order to keep its environment in equilibrium, about 60 percent of the land of a mountainous country like Nepal should be covered in forest. The present rate of deforestation in the country is far beyond the capacity of the forests to regenerate themselves, and this is leading to severe environmental problems.

Thus, poverty and the environmental problems it has caused have both led people from the rural areas to migrate to urban areas of Nepal and India in search of employment. The 1991 census showed that nearly 4 percent of the population had migrated seasonally to India. Prior to 1992, it was observed that most of these migrants were male. After 1992, however, it was observed that a growing number of illiterate women were also migrating to India. This is the principal reason why relatively few young women are seen in some of the villages outside Kathmandu. Reportedly ten thousand Nepali girls are annually trafficked to Indian brothels and it is estimated that in Bombay (India) alone there are about 45,000 Nepali sex workers.

These women who are involved in prostitution, often unable to impose on their clients the use of protective means against sexually transmitted infection, are highly vulnerable to HIV/AIDS. Similarly, migrant males, who have left their wives and families to find work outside the country and who purchase sexual services, are equally vulnerable.

Poverty has contributed to the environmental degradation, in particular deforestation and the erosion of arable land. In turn, environmental degradation has caused a forced economic migration. This unfortunate chain of events has resulted in a soaring increase of the vulnerability of both men and women to the most serious health crisis of our time: the HIV/AIDS epidemic.

Ganesh Gurung, Anthropologist
Consultant, International AIDS Program
Harvard School of Public Health

REFERENCES

Moddie, A.D. "Himalayan Environment," in Lall and Moddie (ed.), *The Himalayan Aspects of Change*, New Delhi, Oxford University Press 1981.

The Kathmandu Post, 5 June and 18 December 1995.

Central Bureau of Statistics Nepal Census 1991.

World Development Report, "From Plan to Market," The World Bank, Washington DC 1996.

"We went into Nepal with the assumption that the calendar was our enemy. That every day we didn't get something done, somebody's life would be on the line. We had a moral commitment to the communities and to AIDS prevention. We were willing to be flexible and responsive and not to hold all the reins. If you can't share responsibility, you can't do the job. And we had good partners."—REV. MARGARET REINFELD, FORMER DIRECTOR OF AMFAR INTERNATIONAL PROGRAMS

CHAPTER 2

GENESIS OF THE AMFAR RESPONSE
TO HIV/AIDS IN NEPAL

 Since its founding, AmFAR has responded to the HIV/AIDS epidemic with a focus on research objectives in basic science, clinical research, prevention and ethics. In 1989, AmFAR added an international prevention program and Nepal was chosen as a participant in 1993. "Our objective," says former Director of International Programs Rev. Margaret Reinfeld, "was to see if you can get into a country ahead of the epidemic and build a backfire to forestall it. We wanted to work from the ground up with truly indigenous agencies a) to develop their capacity at ground level, b) to develop networks of people at the macro community

level with the capacity to respond to however the epidemic developed in that country and c) to foster government/NGO involvement so the government could see that sector as a way to approach the epidemic in the most sustainable way." AmFAR's research mission is to implement this program model and study the responses to the epidemic that develop out of it: Are they appropriate and effective in the country's context? What lessons can be learned from the perspective of the donor, the NGOs, the communities? Do those lessons have relevance beyond the country's borders?

AmFAR's model called for funding indigenous organizations for three years and providing them with the technical assistance needed to develop their organizations to a level that made their HIV/AIDS program sustainable. A request for proposals was advertised throughout Nepal. "We analyzed 80 applications for their links to the community and their potential, not for their track record," says Rev. Reinfeld. "Then we funded 17 of them with the commitment that, after the first round, funding would be non-competitive. That meant they were free to make mistakes, share information." The NGOs selected varied from small budget community based organizations that had formed specifically in response to AmFAR's request for proposals to large, Kathmandu-based service organizations with several years of experience and a range of existing programs. As was expected, none had previous experience in the field of HIV/AIDS.

The wide ethnic and geographic range of the NGOs and the communities served proved to be unique. Nepal's capital, Kathmandu, had always been the center of NGO activity, says anthropologist Ganesh Gurung, "so, when AmFAR funded NGOs right from eastern Jhapa to the west end, the NGOs felt this was a new approach. Before, remote groups never imagined they would get a project. Now, they thought, even though we are not in Kathmandu, we are in the right place. Many Kathmandu NGOs have started district offices in the east and west now, and AmFAR has given an example to other NGOs to go outside of Kathmandu also."

BUILDING A PARTNERSHIP: THE ROLE OF TECHNICAL ASSISTANCE

It was clear to AmFAR from the outset that in order to test the AmFAR model and build the NGOs' capacities, close donor/NGO collaboration would be vital. The key to this is AmFAR's technical assistance program. It provides the NGOs with access to resource people from AmFAR in New York, the Harvard School of Public Health (the AmFAR-contracted evaluation team) and a Kathmandu-based technical assistance staff. "AmFAR never acted like a funder," says Rev. Reinfeld, "we acted like a programmer and designed the program in common purpose with the grantees and treated them like partners. We were intimately involved from the beginning, which most funders can't do because they don't have AIDS expertise. It wasn't up to us to tell the grantees how to develop programs, it was up to us to listen and give them the resources they needed and facilitate, not direct."

Initially, AmFAR contracted with Save the Children/US to provide technical assistance. SCF/US has had long-standing involvement in Nepal and its focus on community development and capacity building seemed compatible with AmFAR's aims and goals. Despite the partial overlap in missions, it soon became clear to both organizations that while some expectations were being met, others were not. Although the relationship between AmFAR and SCF/US did not continue, valuable lessons were learned. Keith Leslie, Country Director of SCF/US feels that many of the problems stemmed from not allowing sufficient time for planning: "If you're going to put in a nationwide program, you'd better spend the first six months just getting to know all the organizations you're working with. There was not enough clarification of job role and what the goal of the program was. Because in AmFAR, which we found out later, there was a great emphasis that this should be a research project. And our sense was, look at these NGOs, look at the situation in Nepal. I don't think any of us realized how much these organizations needed in terms of capacity building. And administratively, it became much bigger than we ever imagined, because of the requirements of AmFAR. In a way, it was better to separate, but it was unfortunate. We all gave a lot of energy, a part of our lives to it."

AmFAR established its own technical assistance agency at the beginning of the project's second year. Five staff members worked directly with the 16 NGOs whose funding was renewed. They spend the majority of their time in the field. "We made an effort when we started out," says Technical Advisor Dr. Paul Janssen, "to go to the remote, community-based organizations first rather than to the ones in Kathmandu. It was a signal that everyone is equal. Especially in a situation like this, where two cultures come together and we know we perceive objectives differently, making those objectives explicit and planning your activities and expected outputs should be an important part of working with the NGOs from the outset."

Both the NGOs and the technical assistance staff have been breaking new ground as they work together. As Program Manager Azeliya Ranjitkar points out, "There is no equivalent in Nepali to 'technical assistance,' not in the language or the culture," and sometimes Nepali culture can complicate the task. "For example, we need to discuss problems together with the NGOs, but in Nepal, you are considered not good enough for a job if you show a weakness, so you ignore problems and there is no incentive to find a solution. Our word for 'supervisor' means 'inspector.' Someone who only finds mistakes and criticizes. The NGOs are just now learning to see us as people who want to work with them to overcome problems. But they *are* learning how to use us, and that means the staff needs to be able to fulfill the NGOs' expectations. It works both ways, and development of the staff is just as important as giving skills to the NGOs. We are all on a learning curve with this."

None of the technical assistance staff had done HIV/AIDS work before, though all had previous experience in community health or development, or NGO training or support. Focusing on HIV/AIDS work has sometimes meant that they must examine their own assumptions and attitudes and learn to work effectively in new contexts. Program Officer Ganesh Shrestha, for example, had never knowingly spoken to a sex worker before. "Initially I felt some agitation dealing with them, but that changed. At first, I thought they would be open and talk to me, but they didn't want to talk about their private life. It was hard for me to ask: 'Why did you become a sex worker?' People don't like that kind of question. Later, I learned to ask it in a better way." Rekha Shrestha, also a Program Officer, says she finds working in the field challenging but rewarding. "I learn from the NGOs. Each one of them is different and has a different approach. I used to be a training officer in my previous job, but we did not learn to reach the grassroots people. To go to the NGO, stay with them for some days, share with them—all of that is new to me. And it is new for them, too. They are psychologically encouraged when we go to the field. They think, 'somebody from the organization is taking an interest in us.' This is unusual."

The role of the technical assistance staff is to guide the NGOs toward recognizing and solving their own problems. "I am a mediator between our organization and the NGO," says Rekha Shrestha, "a person who will help them become aware of something and address it." One of the most difficult challenges for even the most sophisticated of the NGOs has been to understand and accept the usefulness of monitoring and evaluation techniques. Program Officer Ravi Thapa explains how he has worked together with NGOs on this: "Before they started their activities, none of them recorded anything. Hardly any knew how to plan, and delegating responsibility was a problem. Everybody was just planning from one day to the next. What I provided was how to make a detailed implementation plan and monitor their activities. At first some NGOs were only doing the reporting on their activities because the donor was expecting it. They only saw such information as something for AmFAR's research. But after we started doing field visits, they realized these activities benefit them also. I showed them, look, you do financial activity monitoring and program activity monitoring because they are related to each other, you can check if you have enough budget for your activities. Now they monitor and they can take quick action. Three NGOs have already sent a letter this quarter for a budget transfer with their justifications. Before, if someone spent all the budget for IEC materials, they would just stop getting them, even if they needed more. Another good sign is that more and more we are getting requests for specific technical assistance. The NGOs did not often ask for help before. Some still don't understand monitoring, but the ones that do are very confident. The system gives good results without much time—everything is to their advantage."

Not all the NGOs have been equally enthusiastic. But as a report from the NGO WATCH indicates, even organizations that chafe at AmFAR's reporting requirements appreciate its willingness to be flexible, to let them make mistakes and to put them in the driver's seat. "WATCH believes in action rather than doing studies and preparing reports only. WATCH is not a research organization but an action-oriented and willing-to-learn organization. WATCH has always been discouraged rather than encouraged [in] its efforts to initiate and implement participatory processes and innovative ideas; however, it goes to [the] credit of AmFAR that it has been very supportive of our ideas and allowed us to make changes in the program activities as required. We know this has created some problems in terms of monitoring process and achievements."

Along with their work in the field, members of the technical assistance staff also organize skills building workshops for the NGOs and promote development of working relationships among the NGOs themselves and between the NGOs, INGOs and the government. This aspect of their work is discussed in the final chapter.

In addition to reinforcing the lessons of the first year, the technical assistance staff added new focal points in the second year. One is to design prevention activities that more specifically target the sub-populations in the NGOs' communities. Another is to move the focus of monitoring and evaluation away from program compliance toward program quality. "We need to ask questions now like, Who is designing the interventions? Who is identifying the at-risk populations? Who is reaching them?" says Azeliya Ranjitkar. "We should be able to know if they can and are doing the job."

"Our technical assistance component is very different from what we've seen in global programs," says Rev. Reinfeld. "It's very hands on, capacity-oriented and not organizational-oriented. These are Nepalis working in Nepali style. We made the decision not to expect high levels of development or bureaucracy, just the minimum amount of organization necessary to function sustainably. It's been successful for us and needs to be adopted more widely."

THE HISTORY OF NGOs IN NEPAL

In 1986, when the National AIDS Program began, very few
NGOs had programs on HIV/AIDS, and it is unclear how
many work in that field today. Eighty NGOs applied for the
AmFAR program. Since the introduction of multi-party
democracy in 1990, indigenous NGOs have proliferated in
Nepal for several reasons: First, the new democracy created a
more favorable climate for community-based organizations.
Before, NGO-like organizations such as family planning had
been established and sponsored by the government and
were often chaired by members of the royal family. Second,
establishment of the Social Welfare Council as Nepal's NGO
coordinating body ended a period of perceived patronage by
and ineffectiveness of its predecessor organization. The
number of NGOs registered with the SWC jumped from
around 200 in 1990 to over 7,000 by mid 1995. About 75 percent are based in the Kathmandu valley, and the majority are
supra-community organizations led by members of the
urban elite. However, many community-based organizations
nationwide do not register with the SWC. Third, donor policy
has changed over time from supporting government activities to supporting NGOs. This policy change created many
opportunistic NGOs founded only to attract funds. Recently,
however, decreasing resources, increased communication
among donors, and growing professionalism among NGOs
are all having an effect on combating this problem.

[Excerpted in part from *The Role for NGOs in the Implementation
of the National AIDS Program in Nepal* by Dr. Paul Janssen,
London, 1994.]

"I've seen this AIDS presentation three times. It is told in ways we can understand. I would say it is effective, because after these sessions, when we get together someplace in the shade, we all end up talking about what we heard."—KALIDAS LAMICHANE, FARMER, BAGMARA

CHAPTER 3

REACHING OUT TO EVERYONE: BRINGING HIV AWARENESS TO THE GENERAL POPULATION

 As everywhere, the general population in Nepal is really an amalgam of sub-populations and NGOs have found that their interventions must be targeted with that in mind. Several of the most at-risk sub-populations have been singled out by the NGOs for specific attention, and these are discussed in detail in following chapters. But, as many NGOs have found, it can be hard to assign someone to just one risk group, especially in a society where much is hidden. A village woman may also secretly sell sex. A village man may go to sex workers, deny his daughter access to health care or migrate to India if his crops fail. And, given all the hardships they face, both of them may have a hard time believing HIV is much of a threat.

The NGOs have found that gathering information on the literacy and income level, health status, attitudes, values and behavior, of a local population is crucial to designing successful interventions for this target population. NGOs say it is simpler to work with homogenous communities where economic disparities are less visible than it is to target heterogeneous communities where traditional hierarchies of caste, class and ethnicity hold sway. However, the NGOs have found that it is not as effective for HIV prevention in the long run. Working with different ethnic groups separately can create unwanted conflicts in a community, and the success or failure of the intervention programs, the NGOs feel, depends upon the ability to resolve or transcend internal conflicts such as party politics, institutionalized inequities, family relationships, quarrels over water, livestock, or access to facilities.

RISK BEHAVIORS AMONG THE GENERAL PUBLIC

To date, almost all known cases of HIV in Nepal have been transmitted from male to female and female to male. Very little is documented about sexual behaviors in Nepal, but having multiple partners is common, especially for men. Men from all walks of life go to sex workers, often frequently, and while this is considered normal, it is rarely admitted to at home. Women have little knowledge of their husbands' behavior and very little influence over it. Many women assume their husbands are faithful while acknowledging that "men" in general are not. If a man wants to take an additional wife, the search may first involve sex with a number of candidates. A few women, particularly those whose husbands are away working for long periods of time, may have sex with other partners.

Only about 3 percent of couples of reproductive age use condoms, and condom supply and accessibility remain a problem, particularly in rural areas. STD rates are high, and while men tend to seek treatment, women usually do not due to shyness or fear of stigmatization. In one NGO's study, only 40 percent of women surveyed sought treatment for STDs.

As in other Asian societies, in Nepal homosexuality is considered abnormal behavior and is both hidden and ignored. Men in Nepal do have sex with men, but the fact is largely overlooked. Sex is defined by most people as something between a man and a woman, and so by definition, homosexual sex is not sex. Males are reportedly available to both male and female tourists for sex in Nepal. (It is difficult to distinguish between "casual" and "commercial" sex in these cases.) Male children living in Kathmandu's streets told one researcher that they intentionally attract foreign tourists and understand the concept of homosexuality.

Risk of HIV transmission by transfusion has been reduced in Nepal, and 95 percent to 100 percent of the blood supply is reported to be screened. However, several common practices do increase the risk of exposure to HIV in blood. Patients often insist that their medications be administered by injection, which is considered more effective than oral delivery. Re-use of unsterilized needles and syringes is common due to lack of supplies, sterilization equipment and/or fuel.

REDUCING THE RISKS

"Most especially, people always ask me if I can get WICOM to take the program to their village. But usually, that's far away. I feel bad that I can't do what my friends ask, but I can't."—*Lal Singh Tamang, factory peer educator, Pokhara*

INFORMING AND EDUCATING: Interventions to reduce risk for the general population include information/education/communication (IEC) on HIV/AIDS and on a range of related topics (sex and sexuality, general and reproductive health), access to STD diagnosis and treatment, condom promotion and distribution and counseling. Especially effective interventions to date include certain awareness-raising measures, particularly street drama, and condom promotion when it is integrated with family planning activities.

IEC: The universal appeal of street drama—Nearly all of the AmFAR partner NGOs have found street drama to be effective for presenting and perhaps for reinforcing HIV/AIDS education messages. In the first year, many organizations supported their own large troops or hired players. In year two, ten NGOs trained with WICOM and their affiliated drama group, Sarwanam, to establish or streamline their own approach.

"It is extremely easy to draw a crowd in Nepal. If something is going on that looks interesting, people just come up. People who would never stop for HIV information will stop for a drama—it is well adapted to the culture. Nepali people feel it is important share information with others. After our program, someone always asks us if we can go to their village. The men feel they have access to information in Kathmandu, but that the village has none. Some people think of HIV as a rich man's disease because they think it comes from Bombay and Bangkok. Street drama can open dialogue on misconceptions like this and on sexuality in general. It can put the message in the mouth of characters who are like local people.

"Our group uses only one script because the IEC committee has not yet approved the others we have submitted. We know it would be best to tailor the dramas to local audiences and include local themes. What we do now is make minor changes based on audience response. For example, with more educated populations, we add a doctor character who gives more detailed HIV/AIDS information. People see the drama as entertainment and will watch whenever they can and can learn something every time. For example, even after three times, some old men were still saying, 'This is good for the young generation, not for us.' They thought it was only about sex. Then someone said, 'You still get shaved everyday, don't you?'"—*WICOM*

IEC: Tailoring print materials to the community—Early in their programs, NGOs realized there were few, if any, appropriate print materials available for their literate target populations and that other target populations were either illiterate or spoke a language other than Nepali. Some NGOs responded by developing new materials and sharing them with other NGOs. A few problems resulted. It developed, for example, that materials designed for injecting drug users were inappropriate for factory workers. It became apparent that some centralization was needed to make sure accurate, appropriate and non-contradictory messages were being given and to avoid duplication of effort. A standing IEC committee was formed with representatives from several NGOs and advisors from the technical assistance staff.

"One of the first things we learned was that the Tamang, Magar, Danuwar and Tharu communities we target are mostly illiterate and were unable to understand our leaflets and charts. So we started NFE classes, but also we are always responding to feedback about IEC materials we developed. For example, one picture on a poster was a silhouette of a man and woman embracing. It was to indicate sexual transmission. The community said they could not recognize these black figures, but it was the suggestiveness they were objecting to. In the next publication, we changed it."—*WOREC*

IEC: Peer educators and their communities—Whether working with the general population or particular specific communities (the so-called target groups), the NGOs have come to understand that an effective core of peer educators is an invaluable resource, but learning to train them and use them most effectively can be a process of trial and error.

"It is very hard to work in my own village because while we are talking about AIDS, we should talk about sex and sexuality, too. But our taboos say I can't do that openly, especially in front of my sisters and nephews—who have been at the presentations. It is easier in other villages." —*Gopi Raj Adhikari, WICOM counselor, Pokhara*

"Originally, we thought our 12 peer educators could cover the whole Jhapa district, but we realized it is illogical to have someone work far from their residence. Now we concentrate on the six VDCs they are from. 'Peer' here means peer of the general population, which is mixed Bahun/Chhetri and the local Jhapa inhabitants, Tharu, and so on. Our peer educators are from all these groups. They go from house to house in teams, usually one male and one female. They are from the place they work and that is important because with STD work you have to spend a lot of time networking in the community. You can't just walk in and expect people to come to you for treatment." —*B.P. Memorial*

"A major thing that has impressed the people in Nuwakot and Udyapur is that the education on STDs and AIDS has been given in their own languages, Tamang, Magar and Danuwar. Poverty among them is linked with prostitution, and many of their daughters have been trafficked. We try to create awareness about that and HIV. If WOREC staff from Kathmandu went there, people would be shy with us, but they are open with the village level educators, who are local people.

"In AIDS education, we found that different communities learn at different rates. We had more success with our awareness programs in Udyapur than in Nuwakot where the village level educators and the people were not so literate. That little bit of education made a difference, we found. If the educator has less education, he cannot perceive the message as well and cannot communicate it to the community as per requirement. And if the community is illiterate, it is more difficult to understand these things. People from better educated communities present and understand the information better. The first year, we trained all the educators together. This year we have separate training that keeps in mind their education level. But our job is not to send elite Kathmandu teachers out there to explain to them what they need. Our job is to train the local community, and integrate them into society. Although the impact in Nuwakot is slow, there is positive impact."—*WOREC*

PROMOTING CONDOM USE: Nepali condoms are of good quality and meet WHO quality guidelines, but both price and finding a consistent and accessible source have limited their availability, sometimes seriously. At the beginning of their programs, many NGOs found they could not procure large numbers of condoms. One organization could acquire only 300 of the several thousand it had anticipated distributing. This problem was reduced when arrangements were made with a national distributor to coordinate with the NGOs. Far larger barriers to condom acceptance are that people from every walk of life are overwhelmingly shy about discussing such matters, and condoms are distrusted as a family planning method. Condom promotion has been especially difficult among women and conservative ethnic groups.

"I saw the condom demonstration before and I think those villagers who refused to see it today should be convinced not to be embarrassed, because when we saw it, we liked it and learned things we never knew before. In a village like this, the young men have condoms with them, so it is important for them to know how to use them the right way." —*Kalidas Lamichane, farmer, Bagmara*

"It is extremely difficult to tell the Tharu villagers about condom use. They are very shy. Both the boys and girls just walk away. Some men may come and ask us privately for a condom when we go to the village, but never girls or women. It takes maybe three visits, one a month, to establish enough rapport just for females to talk more freely and maybe ask questions. We have no idea how long it will take before they can actually ask for a condom."—*SAFE*

"We have been able to build a lot of trust and rapport in our target area during the first year. We only began distributing condoms the second year at our office and from community workers in the Tamang villages. Most of the takers are men. But also many housewives who think their husbands are not staying just with them."—*MANK*

"We have 20 motivators who cover a 70,000 population house to house with information on HIV and STDs. We have found that if we conduct these health education programs along with family planning programs it is better. Then it is easy to motivate people, especially the hidden sex workers who do not come to us for condoms easily. In a family planning program, the female motivator can easily give out condoms and any woman can easily take them. And if she uses them, we can prevent STDs and AIDS also."—*ICH*

"People are reluctant to use condoms, perhaps because they do not have faith in them. The failure rates are very high because they learned about condoms from family planning workers whose demonstration is not very good. The instructions are vague, they do not go step by step. So we stress that if you use it properly, a condom is very reliable. But there must also be a practical demonstration, ideally individually or in a small group. And also, both the clients and the peer educators are most comfortable with their own sex. In a large group, even our peer educators have problems demonstrating condom use. The mother-in-law, other relatives, respectable persons may be present. Some people just walk away from the group when they see condoms on the flip chart in a demonstration. We make sure they know the peer educator can meet them in private."—*B.P. Memorial*

PROVIDING HEALTH CARE AND STD TREATMENT: The people of Nepal face severe health problems, among them STDs, which are associated with increased risk for sexual transmission of HIV. In year one of their project, some NGOs held mobile health camps where STDs could be detected and treated and at-risk populations could be reached with counseling and education. The camps proved to be both popular and, from the perspective of delivering HIV/AIDS information, problematic. NNSWA has taken a different approach. They do STD examinations and treatment at several rural clinics and also provide HIV/AIDS counseling at a local government hospital's STD clinic. In both settings, they stress the need to go to the government hospital for STD treatment and STD cases at that hospital are said to have dropped dramatically. NNSWA emphasizes the effectiveness of such NGO/government cooperation.

"The first year we did six health camps offering all services, even simple surgery. You cannot imagine it—people would line up at 4 AM. But that was very expensive, so we concentrated on STDs, though we still said 'general camp.' If we said 'STD Camp,' no one would come. We educated all the people who attended about HIV, but only for an hour or two. Follow-up was impossible, also for the STD treatment, because people came from all around. In Nepal, STD diagnosis takes time and we were 40 people seeing 400 people a day. You need to ask a lot of questions in private. People are very shy, especially the women. If she complains of low back pain, we look for an STD. That would be a symptom she could freely mention. Many women go without STD treatment, and just live with the symptoms.

"Now we have an STD clinic where people are referred by our outreach workers or can come in on their own. If you ask the people, they would say they still want the camps. Even though their primary problem is not HIV or even STDs, they understood these as the clear focus of the camps. We realized, however, that the camps were not serving their intended purpose. Now we offer laboratory tests, diagnosis, treatment and HIV/STD education and counseling for 10 Rs per visit—a private doctor would charge 70 Rs—and our outreach workers can do follow-up. But the service is very underutilized. There were only 40 clients in the first month, all referrals. To increase use we have to bring in supportive services, just a few, otherwise, even though we don't call it an STD clinic, people may feel stigmatized. Another problem is the rumor that we deal only with AIDS patients. You see, private doctors have a practice with some pharmacists after hospital hours. The pharmacist may tell a patient, 'Don't go to that AIDS clinic. Wait here for the doctor.' We plan to meet with local doctors and pharmacists and at least urge them to send people to us for health education and counseling after they treat them.

"We need a good relationship with pharmacists, they are the ones who dispense most of the drugs. We also plan to train paramedics at local health posts. When you network widely with the community, it can help you make important changes. For example, an Indian quack was giving shots without sterilizing the needle. One of our peer educators saw this and explained the dangers, but he refused to change. She explained the problem to influential people in the community who told others and together they put a lot of pressure on the practitioner to agree. Now people make sure he sterilizes his needles first."—*B.P. Memorial*

"We established a regular part-time STD clinic at the Tikapur Health Center. But we have difficulty attracting clients, which was not the case when we did STD camps. When we started the clinic people would come and be examined and get medication as well as HIV/STD education. But now we don't have a budget line for medication, and just getting an examination and education doesn't motivate people. They don't take what we do seriously. They say, 'Why are we showing our body to you if we don't get medication?'. It is better to give medication. If we can control STDs we can control HIV."—*ICH*

"We run two general clinics that provide basic primary health care and STD/AIDS education and counseling. If we did not provide general health care, people would not come. They come because there is no medicine at the government health post and the local people know that we have some stock. First our nurses provide education individually or in groups of two or three. Only then do we give medicine. If we provide medicine first, people will leave." —*WOREC*

COUNSELING: In the second year, many NGOs added or expanded a counseling component in their programs, seeing it as key to long-term behavior change for individuals and to changing community attitudes and misperceptions about HIV/AIDS. However, the concept of counseling is new in Nepal. People are unaware of how to use the service and most of the few clients to date have focused on awareness raising rather than on issues of behavior change. The NGOs feel that before it can be an effective tool, counseling must first become acceptable and understood. But counseling has already proven than it can be integrated successfully into the context of Nepal. WICOM learned that although Western style couples counseling does not work in Nepal, if the man's mother is also present to influence her son and speak for her daughter-in-law, progress can be made.

"Counseling is a very difficult job and there must be deference to the clients. And you have to motivate people to ask questions—especially women. For example, if they have questions about condoms, they have to overcome two reluctances, one against seeing a condom and the other against asking a question. We introduced counseling at our office because it would give better, more private service, but we have to create the demand for it. Only six men have come in the two months since we started, four of them since we recently started a publicity campaign."—*WICOM*

"Counseling is not just something people come into the clinic for and then go home. It happens in the field and we find it takes a lot of time. I am not talking about changing risk behavior but about awareness, attitudes. For example, one of our community outreach workers was describing the symptoms of STDs. A woman in her sixties who was having a vaginal discharge was suddenly afraid she had AIDS. Her family brought her to the clinic and we tried to convince them it was a treatable STD. It took three months of counseling and visits before they believed she did not have HIV. They had sent her to live in a separate house, but eventually let her come home. People get sensitized to be aware of HIV and STDs by the education we make available, but they don't always understand completely. We have to explain again and again. I don't know how to prevent these problems in the future—just keep explaining.

"In the matter of counseling for behavior change, we have learned that not all AIDS educators are suited to be counselors just because they know the information. Only peer educators who can demonstrate neutrality should move on to become counselors, and not all of them have that skill. We found role play effective for teaching about counseling. For example, when one educator had to play a counselor, she was imposing ideas she learned as a family planning worker—use the condom like this, dispose of it like this. She was not exploring the client's motives for not using a condom. She is also unmarried, and was very reluctant to demonstrate a condom. We said, we will sit here until you do it—no lunch, no dinner. She did it, but not with the inner drive you want to see when you give a demonstration. Also, she is different from most of the target population—socially and politically active with many connections. To give those who didn't develop the skills for counseling at the beginning another chance, we posted them at the clinic with someone who performed well so they can learn from each other while they do the education. After we evaluate them again, we will see where we assign them to work."—*B.P. Memorial*

THE CONTEXT OF VULNERABILITY

In the first 18 months of their programs, the NGOs have successfully raised HIV/AIDS awareness among their communities, have been challenged by the problems of promoting, demonstrating and distributing condoms, and have begun to develop more comprehensive counseling services to address the question of behavior change. But experience has shown them that even when all these risk-reduction services are present, it is not enough to achieve the desired impact. The societal and environmental factors that heighten vulnerability for Nepal's general population (rather than for specific targeted communities among them) are detailed in Chapter 1. The NGOs are aware that combinations of these factors are leading increasing numbers of people to adopt risky sexual behavior in order to ensure economic survival for themselves and their families. This applies particularly to migrant workers and sex workers. Recognizing this, the NGOs have introduced programs that they feel can address some of the contextual forces that increase risk-factors such as illiteracy, poverty and the particular vulnerability of females.

VULNERABILITY REDUCTION: GENERATING EDUCATION AND INCOME

"You have to look at AIDS together with other problems faced by indigenous people."—*DSS*

Several NGOs have initiated non-formal education programs and income-generating projects as interventions to reduce vulnerability among the general population. MANK and WOREC also include women's leadership training as a way to combat the effects of the low status of women in Nepal, and both organizations see this leadership base as potentially pivotal for future HIV/AIDS work in their communities. Working on an even deeper contextual level, BASE, for example, focuses on issues of legal and human rights and has integrated HIV/AIDS education into existing rights-based programs designed to empower the Tharu community.

NON-FORMAL EDUCATION: Several NGOs provide NFE classes in rural Nepal. BASE works with the Tharu community, which is among the most economically disadvantaged populations in Nepal. BASE has had a very ambitious NFE program for this community for several years and has trained the facilitators to integrate HIV education into the program. Many NGOs find that their NFE classes are popular and well attended, others have encountered problems, usually time constraints, that have lowered attendance. Some NGOs learned that classes should not be held during the agricultural growing season because people, especially those who had to walk a long way to class, had no time to attend. When attendance is stable and facilitators are well trained, NFE appears to provide both a foundation for future empowerment and an effective forum for introducing HIV/AIDS information.

"I chose to go to NFE because I wanted to learn something. My father didn't force me. I went because I saw others going, but I wasn't just copying them. We didn't know about the alphabet and now we do. We know about health and forest fires and AIDS. Now, if the words are easy, I can even read signs."—*Teenage Tharu boy, Chyama Chisapani*

"When we went to the field with NFE for the Badi community, others wanted it too, so now we take it to Tharu villages nearby. Offering this for everyone avoids discrimination. NFE is a good program for the Tharu. If we just did street drama and education, that would focus directly on HIV, but NFE can give broad information on health—water quality, sanitation—things they don't know. It can also give them a chance to say they can read and write, and just that alone can improve their life."—*SAFE*

"We hold NFE classes for males and females from 15 to 45 years of age in two Tamang villages. The class is two hours every evening for six months. The rest of the year people are busy with farming and it is the monsoon. We don't say, we are going to give you lectures on HIV and girl trafficking—no one would come. We say, we are teaching you to read and write. People want that. Then we integrate HIV information into the middle of the class period. Also, each class has a committee that takes what they have learned back to the village. Motivation is high. Only three of 42 did not go on to a second year.

"At first, we had trouble finding facilitators to teach the class because almost everyone was illiterate, but now we have trained 13 of them locally. Some walk all day to get to where they will teach. This area, Sindhupalchowk, is very remote. There is no telephone, no publications. Those not in NFE have a very low chance of exposure to HIV information. For those who have finished the class, our community workers take new IEC pamphlets, comics, whatever they can get, to the villages and people read it out loud and discuss it. But there is not much material available.

"Sindhupalchowk is also a center of girl trafficking and that is a big topic in our NFE classes, and we have truly raised the community's awareness about this problem."—*MANK*

"We conduct ten NFE classes in Udyapur. These are for girls only because we feel they are harder to reach than boys and they are also subject to trafficking. Our philosophy is to empower girls to speak for themselves and we place major emphasis on making them literate. In Nepal, each family sends their boys to school. But in fact, the schools in these rural areas are mostly open in the evening, and often there are no teachers. So even if a boy goes, well, he is there on paper, but after three or four years he is still illiterate. But we are limited in our finances and manpower, so we focus only on girls. Maybe another NGO will extend NFE to boys also."—*WOREC*

INCOME GENERATION: The NGOs have found that developing successful income generation projects for the general population can be problematic. Projects must not only be well matched to the locale and the population, they must also factor in marketing issues and provide enough income to sustain participation. Most NGOs only began these interventions in their second year and although not discouraged, many were surprised at how much more difficult it was to design an effective project than they had anticipated.

"Income generating is not at all simple, it's very, very hard to determine what is appropriate and what is not. It depends on politics, social factors, the personal capabilities of the entrepreneur."—*MANK*

"Our survey of the Tamang people showed that they are trained in bamboo work so we introduced this enterprise along with sewing and knitting training. At first not one household sent their daughter. The Tamang fathers said, 'Why are you asking only our daughters to go to this program? If it was really useful, the higher caste Brahmin and Chhetris would have accepted it first.' They thought, since we did not offer it to high caste people, it could not be a good program. That shows their level of humiliation. Slowly they came, and after six months, there were 64 participants. What changed their minds was the income and the skills generated. When we located the training center, we did not know there was a military camp nearby whose people would buy the clothes and goods. We were lucky they are a good market. I think that if we did not provide any income generating activities along with education and NFE, we could not slow down trafficking. And we have."—*WOREC*

RIGHTS ADVOCACY: Some NGOs are examining the basis of the economic deprivation and low quality of life of the "general" populations they serve, and are finding that denial of human and legal rights may play a large role. While there is some movement among several NGOs to include rights advocacy in their programs, BASE has developed the most comprehensive interventions. BASE's rights-based philosophy seeks to empower the Tharu, among the most disadvantaged people in Nepal, toward community development and assertion of their land rights.

"BASE is a movement for social change. The Tharu people occupied most of the Terai until malaria was controlled in the 1950s. Then many were systematically squeezed off their fertile land by moneylenders and landlords from the hill region. As a result, the majority became landless and were forced to migrate to India or work as bonded laborers. Lack of education was an essential cause of being deprived of land, political and human rights. Our slogan is 'First Focus on Education' and NFE is our largest component. HIV education and education about land and human rights is integrated into the curriculum. But education alone cannot solve the problems, and our programs include other components such as income generation, health, legal aid, HIV education."—*BASE*

LOOKING AHEAD TO FUTURE INTERVENTIONS

Given the general lack of HIV awareness in Nepal, the fact that it has been significantly increased among the NGOs' target populations in so short a time is, in itself, a major accomplishment. But as many NGOs have found, awareness is not behavior change, nor does it address the context of people's lives. There are several areas that may merit study for developing future interventions for the general population.

Most HIV in Nepal will not be diagnosed or come to the attention of the system, and outreach programs will be needed to find, educate and support people with HIV/AIDS. Developing community based support systems may prove to be particularly important, for here, as elsewhere, the burden of care will fall on family members—most often on women who will have to add it to their already heavy work load.

Even for women and men in stable relationships, the nature of gender relations in Nepal can put partners at risk from HIV. More research is needed to see how best to empower women and help develop their communications skills so they can negotiate safer sex with their partners. It would also be valuable to research ways to establish more open communication about behaviors, and ways to define and build on intrafamilial relationships that can influence and guide behavior. NGOs stress that it is important to include in such research development approaches for men as well as women.

Alternate income generating projects for this population have had limited success so far and thought might be given to integrating them into more fundamental approaches to addressing Nepal's poverty. For example, HIV prevention would also be served by a project to reforest highly vulnerable areas as a way to simultaneously generate income and slow out-migration.

Other issues affecting Nepal's general population that may merit more attention include: addressing vulnerable and so far overlooked sub-populations such as homosexual men and workers in the tourist industry; research on interventions to promote needle-sterilization by health care providers; and attention to counseling women about perinatal transmission.

NIGHTS CLASSES IN THE TERAI

The Tharu village of Chyama Chisapani is a tight cluster of clay-plastered one and two story houses an hour by jeep from Nepalgung in the Terai. One of the SAFE educators has described the Tharu to me as "an illiterate and exploited people who work almost as slaves for their landlords." The village leader I meet, however, is both literate and relatively prosperous. A soft-spoken man, he is also an NFE facilitator, and enthusiastic about the program: "The participants are very easy to motivate. That is because the timing is good, from 8 to 10 PM, after chores. At first, the participants felt embarrassed by the AIDS chapter in the book because it tells of sex and condoms. But I told them, this is for us, all humans can get this. That lessens the embarrassment. Now they want to know more." After exhaustive coaxing, a shy teenage girl describes to me (through two translators) how NFE fits into her life: "I know that at my age, lots of people know a lot, but I can't even read. I don't want to miss any of my class. If I can't finish my housework before it starts, I leave it for my ten brothers and sisters and go. Every morning I tend the cattle. Then anytime between 8 and 12 we eat. Then I go out into the fields and work until it is time to come back and help my sister-in-law before dark. Then except for Saturday, there is NFE at night." A teenage boy is far less shy with me, and he only hesitates a little before saying the word condom. "I can read signs now. And before, I didn't know anything about HIV and now I know it's a killer that can come anytime. Now, I make sure the doctor uses a new needle. And in the other matters, well, if I need the information, I'll be aware of how you get HIV. If I ever need one, I'm sure I can use a condom the right way because I saw the video."

Classes begin after dark. SAFE provides training for the facilitators, the services of the field coordinator, and a blackboard, chalk and four kerosene lanterns for each classroom. In the children's class, the facilitator reads a parable about two goats. On a second story terrace, older youths quietly copy out words. In a room nearby, some 25 adults, mostly women, sit on the floor clustered around the lanterns. They move their fingers under the words and repeat after the facilitator. "Always," "Always," "use," "use," "a," "a," "condom," "condom," "when," "when," "having," "having," "sex," "sex." In Nepali, it sounds musical and very hypnotic. This is the way things are taught in Nepal, by repetition and rote memorization. Tomorrow, when the SAFE field worker comes, there will be a focused discussion on tonight's chapter. After listening a while longer, we make our way in the pitch dark back to the jeep. Classes will go on for another hour.

"We think that because we don't speak about sex

in this culture children don't know about it."—*CDS*

CHAPTER 4

BREAKING A CONSPIRACY OF SILENCE: HIV EDUCATION FOR THE YOUNG

The majority of Nepal's population is young, and there, as elsewhere, HIV will be an epidemic of the young. In Nepal, sex and sexuality are typically not discussed in families and there is no education on the topic provided in the schools. Youths get most of their information on the topic from peers or the media, and it is unlikely to be accurate.

As the traditional economy weakens, a growing number of poor and extremely naive youths, male and female, are migrating to urban centers to look for work, although their chances of finding it have been reduced by the recent ban on employing children under the age of 14 years. The number of street children in Kathmandu and some of the larger cities is growing daily and there are very few services for them.

Age at first intercourse for girls is low in Nepal. Child marriage is common, and although the legal age for marriage is 16, almost 40 percent of girls marry earlier, some as young as 13. Boys tend to marry somewhat older. Illiteracy is higher among girls than among boys. In the villages in particular, girls begin helping with household and agricultural chores by the age of five or six, an age when their brothers may already be in school. Only about one girl in three will attend primary school and far fewer will continue on. Most girls work more hours and get less food and access to health care than boys of the same age.

RISK BEHAVIORS AMONG YOUTH

It is safe to say that the high profile of sexuality and sexual experimentation that is typical among young people in most industrialized countries is absent in Nepal. However, no information is available on the actual sexual practices and attitudes of Nepal's youth. Sex workers (SWs) report visits from boys as young as 14 years, but it is not known how common or widespread this is. With far more access to the media than rural youth, urban boys are more likely to have heard HIV/AIDS messages and to know about condoms, but they are unlikely to know how to use them properly. A high premium is put on girls' virginity until marriage, but naiveté, poverty or unequal status may lead to exploitation or trafficking. Thousands of Nepali girls, some as young as 10 years, are trafficked to Indian brothels each year. (A much smaller number of boys are trafficked as well, though not to brothels.) Of

341 SWs surveyed in the Kathmandu Valley, over half were under the age of 21 years and 72 percent had some type of STD.

Drug use among school students has been recognized as a significant enough threat that the police have prepared a drug abuse awareness package for presentation in schools. Urban boys in Nepal are reported to experiment with drug taking behaviors as young as 8 years and with injecting beginning as early as 12 years. The NGO LALS characterizes up to 20 percent of its 800 needle exchange clients as "street children."

RISK REDUCTION INTERVENTIONS FOR SCHOOL AND CAMPUS YOUTH

"We students can help in controlling the AIDS. We can tell our family, our neighbors and illiterate women about HIV/AIDS. We must not hate the AIDS infected people but rather show them love, affection and give moral support. By shaking hands, embracing, using the same comb, toilets, kitchen or swimming pool and mosquito bites the disease is not transferred. If everybody is aware of the above mentioned points and stays in self-discipline, we can do a lot in preventing the spreading of this disease."
—*From an essay by Laxmi Bista, grade 10, Lalitpur*

Nepali youths in school (ages 12 to 16 years) and on campuses (16 to 21 years) are targeted with HIV/AIDS education programs in the classroom during the school year. The primary interventions are based on IEC materials that are introduced by NGO staff, trained teachers and, in some cases, peer educators. According to several NGOs, ignorance on the part of students, parents, teachers and society about HIV and about sex and sexuality in general may be the greatest factor influencing students' risk of HIV infection at this stage in their lives. There is growing consensus that HIV/AIDS education is most effective among school students. Waiting until they are on campus is "too late." Splitting boys and girls into separate groups is considered most effective, but B.P. Memorial has been able to develop a successful presentation for mixed-sex classes. Training teachers as HIV/AIDS educators is seen as desirable but difficult as it can be hampered by prejudices, lack of commitment and low levels of awareness about sex and sexuality on the part of the teachers. Peer group education, on the other hand, has proven quite effective. It was also found that students can be a good vector of information back to their communities. Transmission is best to siblings and friends outside of school, but unreliable to parents.

"We wanted to go into the schools and not just talk about HIV, but build up a base of knowledge about reproductive health. That topic is in their curriculum, but the teachers just skim it or skip it. This sends a message, if the teachers don't want to teach, the students don't want to ask. We found they were much more open with us than with the teacher. I think the reason talk about sex is stigmatized in Nepal is just because people have never had any opportunity to learn about it. It is not that they don't want to talk—males, females, they do talk. But they don't have the right facts. So we are making it a bit more open and giving them the facts. But Nepali people will never talk openly about sex like Westerners.

"We approached 12 schools in Jhapa and they were all happy to accept this training. There was some resistance from teachers at first. One teacher objected to a picture of a condom in our booklet with the message: Use condoms if you have sex with unknown persons. She said it promoted sex with strangers and wanted it to say: Don't have sex until marriage. I asked, 'When you say certain ways are the right way to act. . .is that the way you acted yourself?' It's high time we re-think for ourselves what the laws of society are. We conducted teacher trainings with the objective of having them act as a resource in the school community as well as facilitate our program in the schools. We want them to understand the importance of AIDS education in the school, and the community, and their role in it. But we may rethink the plan because of this problem with objectivity.

"So we were cautious going in, we sat with the students to make sure they were not offended by the materials. We begin with the reproductive system, then talk about communicable disease, STDs, HIV, and we discuss condoms, but do not give a demonstration. It was important to be sure they would not be too shy to participate because participation is an important part of learning. We don't want rote memorization with no tests for comprehension—the way they learn so much else in school."
—B.P. Memorial

"At first, teachers and administrators were reluctant to participate with our education programs. They had very little information on HIV/AIDS and took the epidemic lightly. Even though the program is well established now, we still face opposition from some administrators.

"We use the same curriculum and IEC materials for both the schools and campuses, which the technical assistance agency has said may be a problem. All the classes are mixed, males and females, except the condom demonstrations. Even the married girls have not seen a condom before. In general, girls are always shyer than boys, but we find that if we go slowly eventually female participation becomes about equal with male in the schools. On the campuses it stays very low. Campus girls don't want to talk about sex in front of boys, they are at that age. School students ask real questions and want information. They learn better and retain more than campus students who have a know-it-all attitude. What these campus boys like most is the condom demonstration. Maybe some of them have already been to a sex worker.

"Also there is a learning difference among the communities. In one Newar village, participation was very low, but in a mixed, more urban community of Brahmins, Chhetris and Newars it was very high. In the conservative all Newar community, social attitudes can make it hard to present such taboo topics. Also they may have trouble understanding Nepali, and we don't give the class in Newar. On the other hand, school and campus students from some of the more remote areas show the most initiative in taking information home to educate their communities."—*ABC/Nepal*

"At first, we put the students above grade eight all together. But the boys did all the talking, so now we have separate groups and the girls do ask some questions. But if the teacher is there, girls won't ask anything! And the boys—their first question is always about masturbation. We make a point of meeting with the teachers beforehand and giving them some control over the program's content, but in the end it is the students' response that determines things. For example, some teachers say it will be bad for the children to talk about sex openly, but when the students come for the education, it is clear that sex is what they want to talk about.

"We think that because we don't speak about sex in this culture, children don't know about it. When teachers and parents learn what kind of questions they ask, it helps them see the need for sex education. When we were worried that the teachers wouldn't give us permission to do the education, we invited all the mothers from one school and showed them the questions children at their child's level had asked. We said, see, if we don't give them education, they will look somewhere else and will probably get the wrong information. Some of them understood quickly. Slowly, slowly, the others also understood, but not in just one session."—CDS

"We don't call what we do bringing the AIDS/STD issue to the school, we call it health education. For example, we would write to a Head Master, 'Dear Sir, we are coming to your school to teach your students about a newly fatal disease epidemic.' Then we are welcomed. First we gave introductory education for the teachers and then trained 34 student leaders immediately after. Then we went to the classrooms and did the education with their help. We have found this two-level training effective and it is a good way to get information back to the village. The education starts slowly, from the beginning. Then later, we come back and talk about AIDS, STDs and so on.

"We discovered that it can be difficult to do the condom demonstration with the model penis in front of students. During the teachers' training it was not a problem. But there were very young girls at the student leaders' training, maybe 13 years old. I tried to do it, but I could not. I asked a supervisor to do it, and he hesitated. Then a Peace Corps volunteer suggested using a banana. So now we demonstrate condoms on a banana for students in 9th and 10th standard. For those younger, there is no demonstration."—*ICH*

RISK REDUCTION INTERVENTIONS FOR OUT-OF-SCHOOL CHILDREN

Children not in school are not only at greater risk than their in-school counterparts, they are also much harder to reach because there are few places where they congregate. Of the AmFAR NGOs, CDS has had the most experience with this population in their work with children in carpet factories.

"In our first year AmFAR program we concentrated on children in the factories because at that time 95 percent of carpet factory labor was under the age of 16. Since then, most of the child workers have been replaced by adults. But maybe up to 20 percent of the labor is still done by children—in factories or at home or in sub-factories. There are also children living with their parents in factory housing, and some are on the streets now. So our original target population has not disappeared, it is just getting harder to reach.

"When we began, we thought that because of the dormitory-like living situation, there was more sex going on than there is. Like other people, we had fixed ideas that there was all this prostitution and the girls were being exploited. It turned out that an older woman will be aamaa—a guardian—to several girls and looks after them. And a lot of the girls live with their parents. So we had to convince them that we were not saying they were at risk because they were prostitutes, but because they were naive. We said, 'You are very young, you come from the villages, you don't know about the city, you can be a target for traffickers.' Slowly we got their confidence. Not by teaching about AIDS, but about life in the city. It was difficult to convince them that they needed HIV/AIDS education and hard to get and keep their attention. Their problems were health and poverty not AIDS. We would talk about anything—movies, make-up—just to get started. Then we slowly introduced AIDS information, but we had to begin with the absolute basics so they had enough background to understand HIV.

"In both the factory and the schools it is easier to get the message across early to separate groups of girls and boys. Younger children listen seriously, but teenage boys just misbehave and the girls are so shy they can't concentrate. In the factory, children just listen at first and don't ask questions until after several sessions. But school children participate right away and ask lots of questions. At around age 13 factory children are not shy about hearing about sex—but only in same-sex groups. We also introduce condoms to children over 13 and do demonstrations."—*CDS*

THE CONTEXT OF VULNERABILITY FOR NEPAL'S YOUTH

"I saw a street drama about girls trafficking. A girl, she got taken to Bombay and came back with HIV. People started talking bad about her. In the time before they took her to Bombay, her life was like my life. This showed me you should not go with anybody. If somebody came and asked me to go India, I'd give him a slap!"—*Suna Lama, 13, Kathmandu*

Interventions to reduce risk among young people have focused on IEC, on sex, sexuality, sexual and reproductive health and HIV/STD prevention. Peer counseling is being developed and expanded, and condoms have been discussed and demonstrated, but not distributed. However, these interventions do not address the contextual factors that increase young people's vulnerability, the strongest among them being the effects of poverty, the taboo against discussing sex and the relative powerlessness of youth. The children of the poor are the most likely to have to work for wages either to help support the family or to provide for their own survival. For girls, this work may include prostitution. Young people who need but cannot find work may face the vulnerabilities common to street children everywhere.

Whether they do not attend school because of poverty or due to ethnic, caste or gender discrimination, illiteracy compounds the vulnerability of out-of-school children. Although a government goal is to provide universal primary education by the year 2000, ensuring girls' participation in these schools will require overcoming tradition, prejudice and an economic situation which depends upon, but does not acknowledge their contributions.

Nepali youths in school and on campus are already in a position of relative privilege. No matter when their education ends, it increases their chance of finding employment, although unemployment is high in almost all sectors of Nepal's economy. For in-school youth vulnerability is increased when authorities seek to "protect" them and decisions about their access to risk-reduction information are largely taken out of their hands. This is likely to happen just as young people are going through physiologi-

cal and psychological changes that they do not understand—
changes that could lead to risk-taking behavior.

INTERVENTIONS TO REDUCE VULNERABILITY

There are relatively few vulnerability-reduction interventions for
youth among the NGOs' programs. The most developed are NFE
classes for out-of-school youth. (Chapter 5 discusses some successful interventions for SWs' children.) NGOs are also working
to develop youth peer counselors and to advocate including sex-
education in school curricula.

NFE CLASSES: CDS conducts NFE classes for the children of carpet factory workers as well as for young people who do or did
carpet work. The parents are generally supportive, although one
father who was affiliated with the Marxist-Leninist party with-
drew his daughters because the text used the example "R is for
Raja [King]." He later realized he was putting the girls at a dis-
advantage and allowed them to return.

"I live with my brother and work every day on his loom. I just
finished my first carpet and hope he will give me 600 Rs for it.
When I don't have to work, I come to study. This is the chapter
we just read about poverty. I thought, this is like my life in the
village. I am just beginning to learn about health from this
book—like if you keep clean, you don't get sick so much. And
now I know how AIDS happens to us, to girls. But the main thing
is to be able to read. There was no money for me to study when
I was small, so now I want to catch up fast. If you don't know
how to read and write, others will discriminate against you."
—*Sharmila Lama, 13, Kathmandu*

"After the child labor act was enforced, the children dispersed and they are harder to reach. Some came to us looking for a place to go. We placed a few, but the best thing we could offer for the others was NFE. Most everyone wants to learn to read and write and NFE might give them a better chance. It is also a good way to incorporate and reinforce HIV/AIDS education. Many of the children who left might never hear about it again, and we think they may be more at risk now than they were in the factories. Also NFE attracts girls, and they are especially hard to reach if they aren't in the factory. NFE can be a basis of women's empowerment. There is a different future for these girls if they become literate." —*CDS*

PEER EDUCATION: An important way to reduce vulnerability for youth is to develop positive peer pressure at school and out of school. This intervention is just being developed, and B.P. Memorial is having considerable success with it in rural eastern Nepal. ABC/Nepal's peer education program in the Kathmandu Valley has been slower to catch on.

"So far students at only four schools out of twelve have shown interest, but we think selecting and training peer educators is very important. Students can't talk with older authority people, but they can ask their peers questions. Also, we know that follow-up activities are a must, but we have found that they can be difficult to schedule before students leave school or go on vacation. It will be easier for peer educators to keep in touch. And that is why the most important thing is to involve the ones who are really interested. You cannot force students to take HIV/AIDS education, so train those with interest and they will train their peers and provide role models." —*ABC/Nepal*

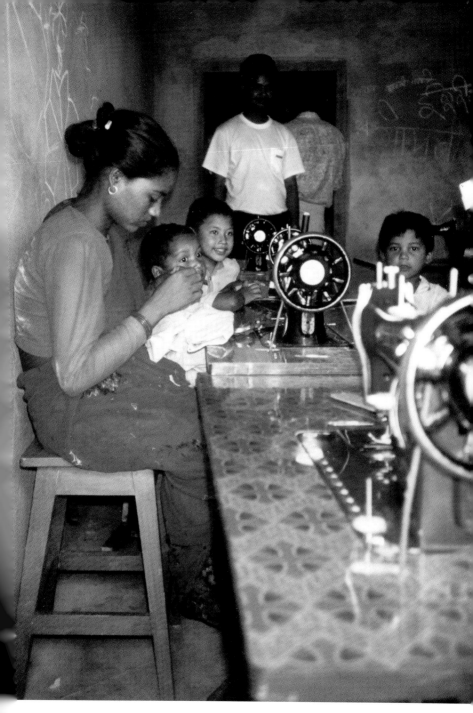

A Nepali woman participates in an alternate income generation program. (Sally Morrison)

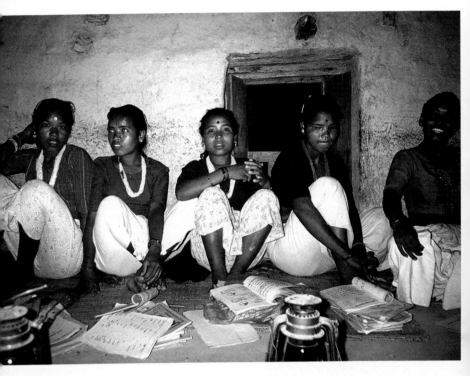

Non-formal education can result in literacy in two years.
(Sally Morrison)

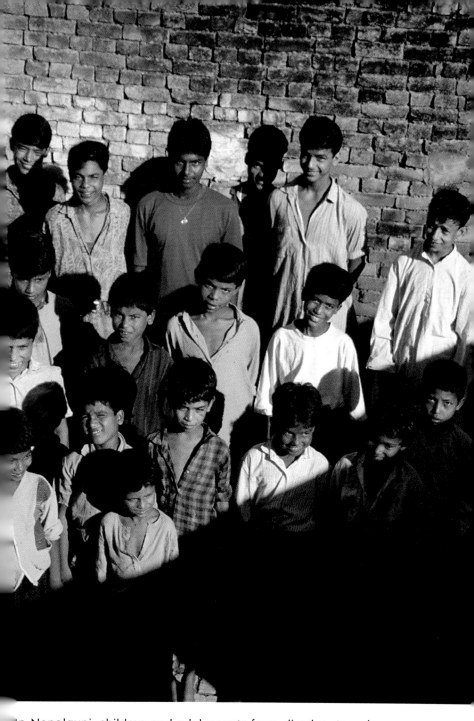

In Nepalgunj, children and adolescents from disadvantaged communities benefit from access to education. (Daniel Tarantola)

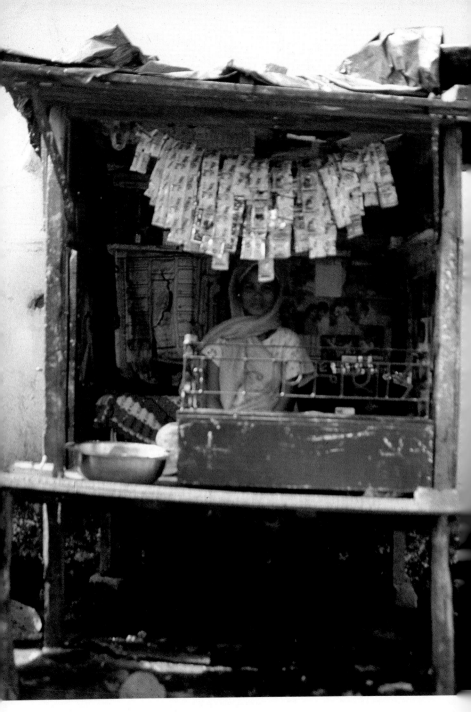

A young woman in difficult circumstances gets a grant to start a small business. (Daniel Tarantola)

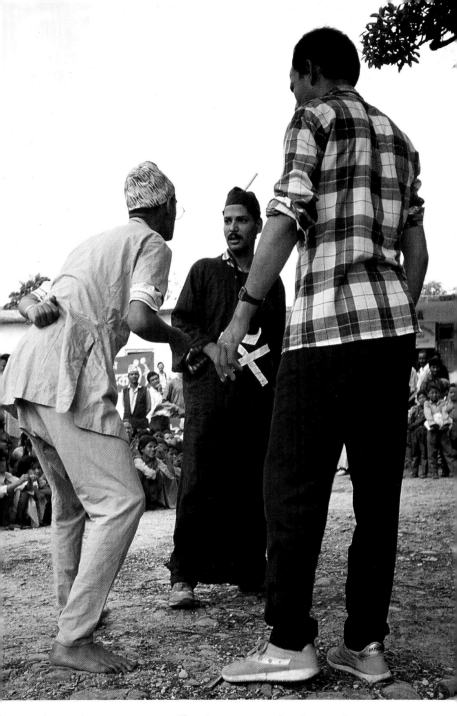

Street drama has proven an effective communication tool
in a community where few can read. (Sally Morrison)

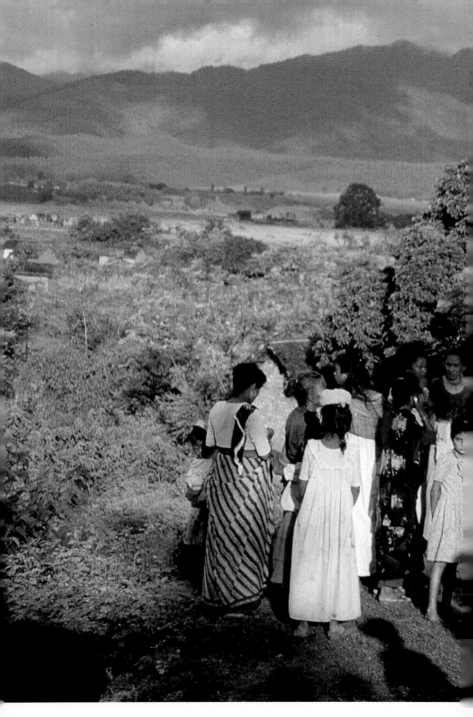

A village community participates in HIV prevention.
(Daniel Tarantola)

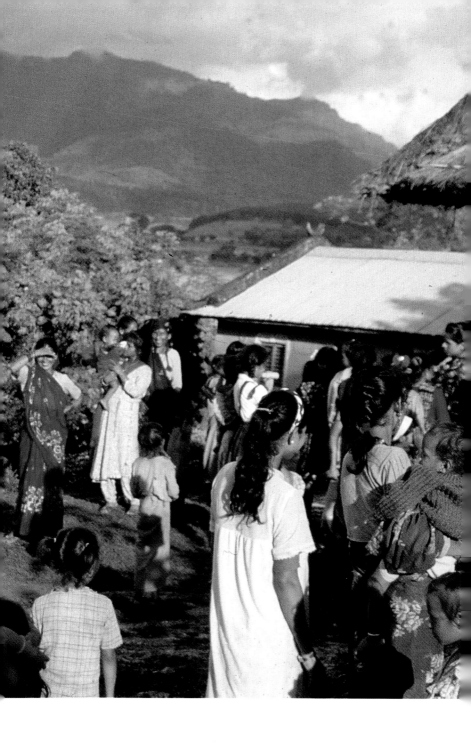

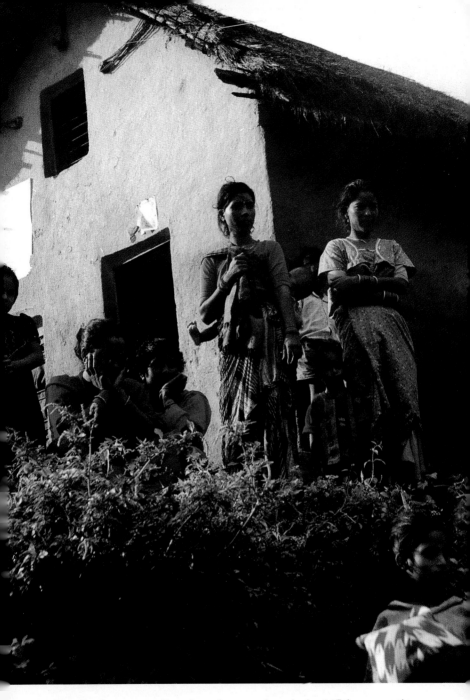

The Badi community played an early role in AIDS prevention programs. (Daniel Tarantola)

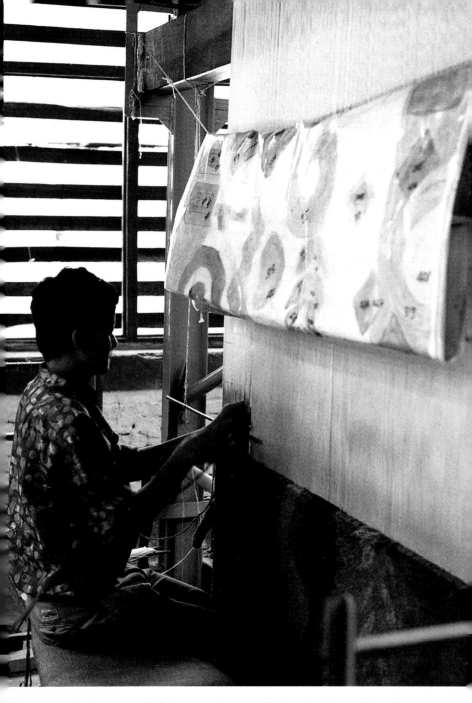

The carpet industry, which is a major contributor to the national economy, employs a large number of migrants in the Kathmandu Valley. (Jill Hannum)

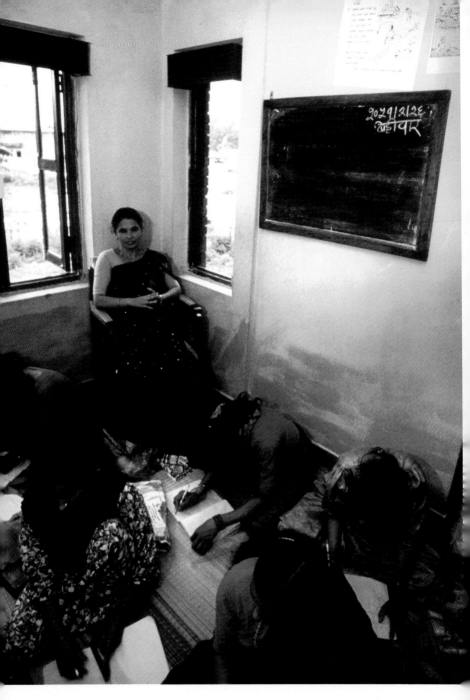

Women who have been marginalized by their villages find housing, training, and support in a community shelter. (Chris Brown)

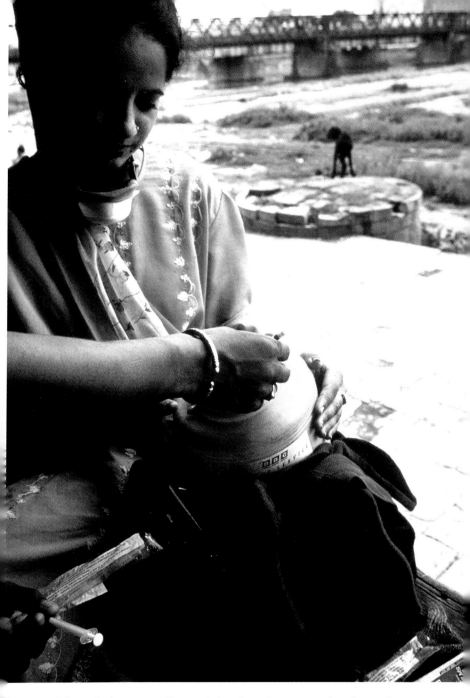

The provision of clean needles to injecting drug users has kept the
rate of HIV infection extremely low in this vulnerable population.
(Chris Brown)

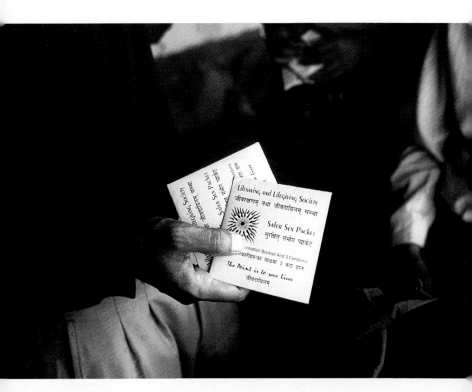

Free distribution of condoms is the first step towards safer sex practices and will later lead to self-sustaining distribution systems. (Chris Brown)

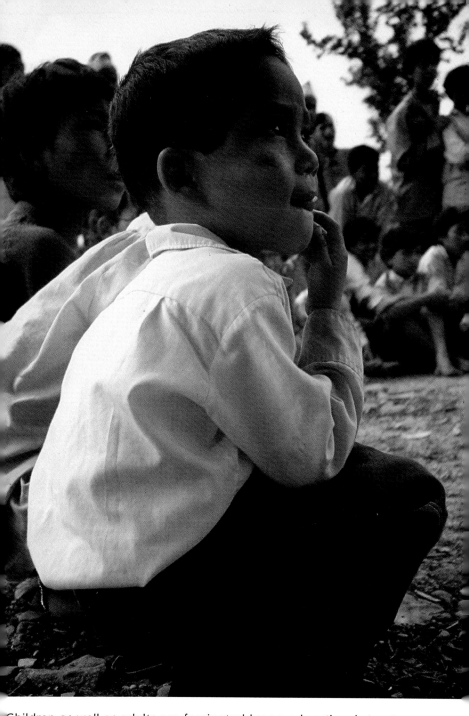

Children as well as adults are fascinated by an educational street drama touring their village. (Sally Morrison)

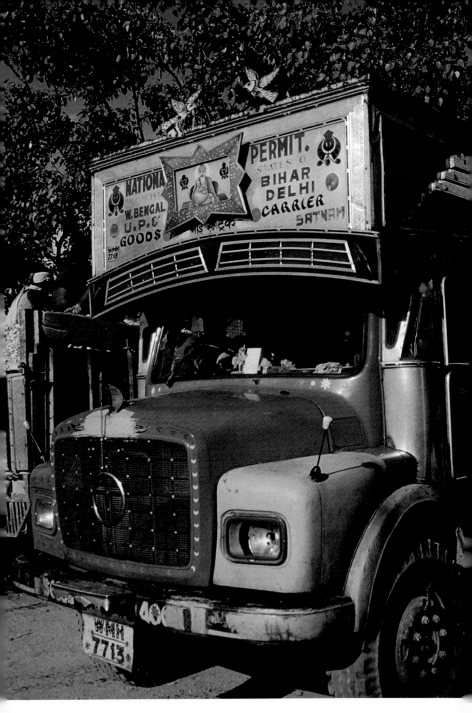

Buses are few and far between in a country where distances are usually measured in walking-days. (Daniel Tarantola)

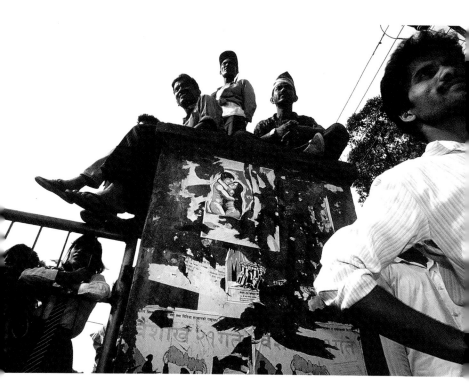

Workers on a break pause to watch when an AIDS education programs comes to their factory. (Chris Brown)

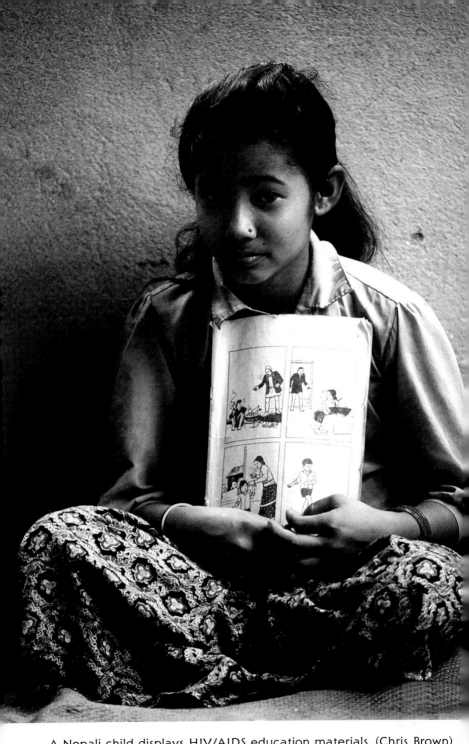

A Nepali child displays HIV/AIDS education materials. (Chris Brown)

"We have developed focus peer groups who will be trained in classroom programs at the schools. This program depends upon a student participatory approach which is essential. Their training will go into more detail than our school education program does. We can also talk with them about the positive aspect of sexuality, not just how you get AIDS and STDs if you have sex. This is not something we can bring to the education at this stage, and the teachers can's do it, but the peer educators can go and talk with others." —*B. P. Memorial*

LOOKING AHEAD TO FUTURE INTERVENTIONS

Increased knowledge about sexual attitudes and practices among youth would help target interventions toward at-risk subpopulations and would also facilitate developing behavior change interventions. NGOs acknowledge that soon interventions for in-school youth will need to go beyond awareness raising to include more controversial elements such as education on sex and sexuality, condom distribution and STD referral. An important next step to facilitate this might be to research effective ways to encourage the support and non-judgmental participation of teachers and administrators, perhaps by involving a broader spectrum of the community, especially parents.

Lobbying to bring sex-education into the curriculum is something NGOs feel is vital not only for facilitating HIV/AIDS education but also for empowering youth. This is a future goal for CDS: "Sex education has to be implemented country wide if Nepal wants to prevent HIV. Maybe you don't call it that yet—you say 'reproductive health.' But it is still a challenge, especially to get it into the schools. How to establish it as a policy, that's a problem. Perhaps get the parents more involved first—the women, the mothers. We have a saying: If you teach a man, you teach one person, but if you teach one woman, you teach the whole universe."—*CDS*

Researching effective outreach and intervention strategies for out-of-school youth and street children may soon become increasingly important. However, there is also a need to advocate for these children's rights and protection, as the accompanying Box on Child Labor details.

CHILD LABOR AND CHILDREN'S RIGHTS IN NEPAL

In 1993, Nepal's carpet industry relied heavily on the labor of children under the age of 14 years and was providing 60 percent of the country's export income. By mid-1994, the industry was rapidly shrinking and the number of children employed had plummeted. The complex linkage between economics and child labor in Nepal provides a cautionary tale for the international community about the impact of a human rights agenda that at first glance may seem straightforward.

Child labor is common and socially accepted in Nepal. The carpet industry began to burgeon in the 1960s, and eventually became the country's largest employer of children. A combination of industry growth and rural economic hardship fostered hiring children as laborers: they needed work and they were obedient. Even more than adults, they were unlikely to assert their rights or leave one factory for another—even if mistreated.

Brought to factories by parents, relatives, or brokers, children comprised a large but never substantiated percentage of workers which according to NGO studies

---

[Based on "Do Laws to Prohibit Child Labor Protect Child Workers in Nepal? The impact of law enforcement on the vulnerability of child workers to HIV/AIDS," by Masumi Watase, Research Assistant, François-Xavier Bagnoud Center for Health and Human Rights, Harvard School of Public Health; 1995 (unpublished report).]

ranged between 11 and 36 percent in the mid-1990s, a range significantly higher than the Ministry of Labor's estimate of less than one percent. The living and working conditions in factories were often dark and cramped and food inadequate. Children were likely candidates for economic and sexual exploitation by adults. Respiratory and eye problems were common occupational hazards; these and many other common health problems generally went untreated.

Until the mid-1990s, the Nepali government had not moved to address these issues, despite NGO pressure to do so. Nepal's Interim Constitution (1950) prohibited the employment of children under 14 in industry, mining or hazardous work, but these provisions were never enforced. In 1990, coinciding with the advent of democracy, Nepal ratified the United Nations Convention of the Rights of the Child. There were soon changes in Nepal's domestic laws, including creation of The Children's Act which established child welfare boards and, among other provisions, reiterated the specific prohibition of employment of children under 14. The act includes provisions for monitoring compliance and punishing violators. Starting in 1994, children under 14 began to be forced out of carpet factories, even though the government had not yet begun to implement the new law. Carpet sales, which had flourished between 1989 and 1994, abruptly dropped off.

A German television documentary that used exaggerated statistics to expose conditions in Nepal's carpet factories seems to have precipitated this response. As buyers canceled about 40 percent of orders from abroad, business continued to drop. Although manufacturers blamed negative press, additional factors were in fact at work: inventories were overstocked because of overproduction; lack of quality-control resulted in declining quality; and there were insufficient efforts by manufacturers to diversify their world market. Consequently, owners of larger factories voluntarily began to discharge their young workers. About half of these factories failed to provide assistance to the now unemployed children, while others helped some of the children to return home. Over time, economic pressure has driven most of them back to Kathmandu where they find themselves in acute competition for work with other former carpet factory children. Their employment opportunities are limited to restaurants, manufactures (including smaller carpet factories), hotels and lodges. A few, mostly boys, have become street children and NGOs report that a small number of girls have turned to prostitution. Without substantial support, coping strategies these children are forced to adopt are likely to have a negative impact on their health and in particular on their vulnerability to sexually transmitted diseases, including HIV/AIDS.

The government does not provide health or support services for these children. Several NGOs run centers for children in transit, but their primary purpose is to reunite children with their families and stays are limited. International concerns such as the Asian-American Free Labor Institute (AAFLI) have focused on the discontinuation of child labor. In early 1995, AAFLI opened a boarding school specifically for young former carpet workers. Although a positive step, future funding and long term sustainability of the ongoing initiative—let alone its expansion—are uncertain.

AAFLI is also working with UNICEF to implement the "rugmark project," which was borne out of a bill passed by the US Congress prohibiting importation into the United States of any goods produced using child labor. In theory, certified manufacturers would be required to pay one to two percent of their sales in exchange for license to use a rugmark certifying no child labor was involved in the production of these carpets. The funds generated by this project would support initiatives intended to benefit the concerned children. The program has not yet been implemented, and its future is in doubt. The government has started its own rugmark program, and there are now so many players that they seem unable to form a coherent vision. Furthermore, industry cooperation remains uncertain. Only a small percentage of manufacturers currently support the program, and success will only be possible with full cooperation. Manufacturers are reluctant to pay the required fee in a time of declining sales, and when their large inventory cannot qualify for the rugmark. From the perspective of helping the unemployed children, the time lag between securing funding from fees and actually implementing programs would have to be measured in years. Finally, as the aim of rugmark is to abolish child labor, it is not clear whether it would have any effect on the improvement of conditions for those children still working or be of significant benefit to children as a whole.

International concern is focused on stopping child labor, and Nepal is one test ground. But the international community remains ill prepared to address consequent issues: Nepal's experience illustrates the complexity of predicting both the long term consequences of, and constraints to, effective discontinuation of child labor.

Confronting these realities, the Nepali CDS observes: "The factory owners think the ban on children working is temporary, and so do we. This is really a question for the government about rights. If you think only in terms of human rights, of course children should not work and it's better for them to be home in the village. If that were possible, they would not have left. The children often told us the situation was better in the factory than at home where they would not get enough food and they sometimes had to work even harder. Under the circumstances, children should be allowed to work, but the conditions should be humane and they should have education and health care available."

CHAPTER 5

PROSTITUTION IN NEPAL: SEX WORKERS AND THEIR CLIENTS

In Nepal sex work is illegal but widely practiced. Sex workers (SWs) are highly stigmatized, yet it is understood by both men and women that "all men" will patronize them if necessary in order to satisfy their sexual needs. Most Nepali women who exchange sex for goods or money do so out of economic necessity. Their clients, however, can represent the entire socio-economic spectrum. It can be very inexpensive to purchase sex in Nepal and it is beyond almost no one's means.

In Nepal, nearly all SWs are female and customers male. Sex workers work anywhere—at home, along major transportation and trekking routes, in urban parks and streets, hotels and broth-els, guest houses and tea shops. Most SWs, whether full-time, part-time or occasional, work covertly and are often referred to by NGOs as "hidden." There are no statistics on their number, although some sources say 10,000 or more. These sex workers come from all ethnic groups and castes and can be found throughout the country. In contrast, an estimated 4,000 Badi women, a caste of traditional sex workers, work openly in their communities in western Nepal. There is also an unknown num-ber of women called Deuki who have been consecrated to tem-ple deities and are said to do sex work at temples. Finally, some 100,000 to 200,000 Nepali girls and women work in brothels in India.

RISK AND RISK-TAKING BEHAVIORS

In some Bombay brothels, 60 percent of SWs are HIV positive. The risk for Nepali SWs in India is high and many of their clients there are men from Nepal—as many as five a day according to one NGO's survey. When these women return home, they may continue their sex work. Of the 331 HIV positive cases docu-mented by October 1995, 134 were SWs and 164 were classified as male SW clients and/or STD patients. A survey of 341 SWs in the Kathmandu Valley found that 72 percent had some type of STD. Although 60 percent were aware of AIDS, only 20 percent reported using condoms most of the time. Three were HIV pos-itive. A survey in the Terai found that only 19 percent of SWs' clients, over half of whom were married, reported using condoms all the time. Their average number of visits to sex workers was four a month.

Sex with a sex worker is not considered to affect a man's virginity before marriage, and some people believe it is not "sex" at all and therefore is not adultery. However some people also believe that only sex with a sex worker can transmit HIV.

REDUCING RISK: SEX WORKERS AS EDUCATORS

Risk reduction interventions targeting SWs and their clients include IEC, STD diagnosis and treatment, condom promotion and distribution and counseling. The success of these interventions has depended largely on which sub-population is being targeted, SWs in a community (the Badi) or the harder to reach full or part time sex workers not in a community.

OUTREACH: Identifying sex workers and gaining their trust and participation in program activities has been a time consuming challenge for the NGOs targeting "hidden" sex workers—these who, unlike the Badi, find it necessary to keep a very low profile to their sex work. The Badi self-identify as a community of common interest, and they had been targeted with NGO programs for several years before AmFAR made it possible to add an HIV/AIDS component to family planning and other programs that had been active in this population.

"I've learned from LALS that I'm at risk from both sides. When you have so much risk...well, before, I might have disappeared. Or I might transmit to many. Yes, I've learned a lot."—*SW/IDU, Kathmandu*

"It is very difficult to identify the first sex worker in a new place, but once it is done she will inform the others about our program.

Identification is easier through the pimps, and we identify the pimps by cultivating the hotel owners. We have also found that the Dada, the local gang boss, knows everything about sex work in his territory. We get a lot of negative comment for working with this man, but we acknowledge his influence. And sometimes he says to us, that girl over there, she works out of such and such a hotel. Then we introduce ourselves to her, invite her to our office and treat her like everyone else. We don't say we think she does sex work, and she may admit it only after many contacts. Also, the girls are hard to contact and follow up with because of migration. We recently expanded from three to eight sites in order to be available in the whole local migration area. Before, we just hoped they would take the education with them wherever they went."—*NESCORD*

"It has been hard for our village peer educators to find out who the sex workers are. One visited a woman's house several times. Because she asked for condoms, he did some follow-up and learned she was one of five women who carried wood to the nearest market to sell. On the way they would do sex work. So, that peer educator lived in that village, and he was aware about SWs and STDs, yet knew nothing of this. You cannot just go to a community, you have to go deep into it many times. There are no indicators for who is a SW. These five women are 35 to 47 years old and their families have no idea they do this. It takes all day to sell the wood and earn 50 Rs. They can get that much in half an hour for sex."—*B.P. Memorial*

"The main thing you need when you are working with SWs and IDUs is networking with other agencies and rapport with those populations. But it's a different, more time-consuming approach with the SWs than with the IDUs. Sex work is even more taboo than injecting drugs. IDUs will talk with us openly in the field, sex workers need a private place. And after five is the best time for contact, but we can contact IDUs at any time. If we had the time to target sex workers, we don't feel it would be difficult to contact them. Some of the SWs also inject drugs—one will tell others about us. That was how we first reached them. Also, we have very good networking. The police used to get several SWs a night and would call us, and our female outreach workers would go counsel them in jail or bring them to the office."—*LALS*

"The police used to harass us and sometimes try to rape us. Once, some of the boys from SAFE tried to protect us from some drunk police and there was a fight. Six men and one girl got arrested. The police demanded a 10,000 Rs deposit to let them go, so we asked everybody for 200 Rs. The working girls gave and households with no girls working sold some things for the money. Everyone contributed. We made this sacrifice because of all that SAFE has done for the community."—*A Badi sex worker, Nepalgung*

"There is much prejudice against the Badi. We cannot educate just them about HIV/AIDS, the whole society has to be involved. The Badi get blamed for bringing HIV into Nepal, even by those who should know better—like one NGO's representative who implied it at a rally near the Indian border. That was damaging and SAFE immediately called a meeting of that NGO, local leaders, police and the Badi to make sure they all got a clear message about HIV/AIDS. Working with such a sensitive issue, everybody has to be clear.

...re we can educate the general public and especially ...cal leaders, social workers, journalists and the police, ... everyone will understand the real risk. At educations we s... ...ss that the Badi are very aware of HIV/AIDS but their problem is in motivating certain groups of clients, like the police, to use condoms. That is when people realize HIV is a general threat. The Badi feel more secure because we do general education. They say it is getting easier to motivate clients and awareness is growing that AIDS is not just a Badi problem.

"If the Badi feel that they are being singled out or pressured to stop doing sex work, they are less willing to participate. Many of us are from the Badi community and we know their problems, but we still had to build trust. First, all of us work very hard for our community and that is noticed. Second, we brought the message in as many ways as we could think of—video, IEC, peer education. It took six or eight weeks to convince them that our message wasn't no sex but safer sex. We also provided things in addition to the HIV/AIDS message that fit their real needs and hopes, like income generation, NFE, a boarding school for the children. Many Badi feel very strongly now that their children should not go into this business. What we do serves that goal.

"Even though we are from the community, we still had to learn from the sex workers. For example, originally, we hired six Badi men to go to the field. But the girls weren't comfortable hearing about condoms from men. Eventually, we found that female motivators who are ex-sex workers are most effective. They can be around the Badi all day. They know the community and have time to work with SAFE. Current sex workers can't spare much time. Recently, we've also begun to involve the sex workers' extended family in understanding HIV/AIDS. Family members who depend on a sex worker financially can be very rude to her if they don't understand. They think, well, if using a condom interferes with her earning, maybe we can't support that. So based on feedback from the community about family pressure, we have started family orientation classes."—*SAFE*

"Twenty-nine Badi households are covered by our program. The number is not very big, but there is a lot of potential for HIV. Kailili is an area of great migration, and many transport workers stay by the highway there. The project staff is from the Kailili region, but not from the Badi community, and we had some problems at first gaining their full trust and support. There was perhaps some level of negative attitude toward sex workers and also a hesitation to talk about sexuality and condom use with them. Two other things also made it hard: the women felt the society was discriminating against them as being carriers of AIDS and they feared legal action by the police. We learned that to be effective, we had to get very close to the target group and give them the right message. The wrong messages got out to the Badi at first—for example, they thought our STD camp only targeted them and they would not come until we made sure they knew it was for the general public, too."—*ICH*

CONDOM PROMOTION AND STD DIAGNOSIS AND REFERRAL: NGOs have had considerably more success promoting condom use among the Badi than among other sex workers. The Badi's personal and economic interests can be addressed directly, and they have a strong internal support network. Nevertheless, many of the lessons learned are broadly applicable."With condoms, we're saving our lives. When we didn't know about condoms, we had STDs all the time. But not any more. We used to have to go to India for treatment, and it costs a lot of money to be in a hospital in India. So we had to borrow that money, and plus, we couldn't earn by sex work when we were sick. So after condoms, we can do our work safely. And we've even begun to have savings." —*Badi sex worker, Nepalgung*

"We have had the most success with condom promotion with Badi sex workers. We stress that this is for self help, for prevention of HIV and STDs. It takes about a month of regular contacts to get them to adopt condom use. Infrequent classes and motivations aren't enough. Unfortunately, within that month they will have unsafe contacts. Also, they often don't use condoms with the partners they trust or have taken as a 'husband.' We have to respect their feeling, but we say, if you are not sure of his background, we know you can motivate him to use condoms when he is with any other partner. The sex workers are quite skilled at motivating now. Before AmFAR, STDs were epidemic here. A doctor checked 40 Badi girls and 75 percent had an STD. We did many referrals and established good coordination with the STD doctor here. But the rate of condom use among these women has increased dramatically, and now the STD specialist says he hasn't seen STDs among the Badis in maybe six months. So the women solved their problem themselves.

"SAFE distributes 8,000 to 10,000 condoms a month, and we have just begun a pilot program of condom social marketing that is proving very successful. We stress self reliance, and if condoms are free, that is not self reliance. Also this system of distribution means there is enough supply, and proper storage and they are available when and where they are needed. That is not something SAFE could guarantee into the future. A test program showed that the sex workers used the same number of condoms per month whether they were free or had to be purchased." —*SAFE*

"A main incentive for Badi women to use condoms is the knowledge itself about AIDS. Before, they knew that they could buy some medicine to stop STDs, but they could not bear the idea of an STD that would cost their life. We found that 90 percent of the Badi women had heard about condoms but they were not using them. The problems were availability and price. Customers who wanted to use them had to bring them. So we made condoms available for free and got a reliable supply. Then we designed a poster to promote condom use. First we put it outside their houses. Then the sex workers suggested that it should be inside their room where it could help educate the clients at the right time. 'You say you don't like to use the condom. See the poster, this is what it promotes and it is the right thing to do.'

"We found that the others, the hidden sex workers, are not coming to us for condoms so easily, but if we conduct our health education programs along with a family planning program, then they can easily take condoms from the female motivator." —*ICH*

THE STIGMA OF SEX WORK

While sex workers are provided with the means to reduce their risk of HIV infection in their professional sexual encounters, their reasons for doing sex work remain largely dependent on the context of their lives, which also has to be addressed: stigmatization deprives them of community support and permits harassment and exploitation by authorities. Poverty often determines the decision to go into sex work, especially now that increasing numbers of women need income to help support their families. Economic need, tradition, ignorance and the low status of females perpetuate the practice of trafficking. Just as they do for women in the general population, gender inequality, illiteracy and naiveté all add to sex workers' vulnerability to exposure to HIV, but with the added risks of multiple partners, and an illegal and highly stigmatized occupation.

ENABLING SEX WORKERS TO REDUCE THEIR VULNERABILITY

Vulnerability reduction interventions for sex workers and women at risk of entering sex work have focused primarily on non-formal education and income generation programs. Women's leadership development programs play a less direct role. NGO's efforts to empower sex workers' communities have generally grown out of responses to immediate needs rather than being developed as planned interventions.

NON-FORMAL EDUCATION: NFE classes are seen not only as having intrinsic value, but also as a vehicle for providing information targeted at sex workers without singling out anyone for stigmatization. Classes designed to attract from the community at large women who are sex workers or are at risk for sex work have generally been more successful than classes targeting Badi sex workers. SAFE, ICH and NNSWA have all found that educating Badi children so they can find alternative livelihoods may be a more effective long-term intervention.

"This is precious time for study and not work. Instead of working 12 hours as usual we can just work 10. It doesn't make any difference if I lose that income. I can be a sex worker for many more years. Right now is the time to learn. And I've learned how to save my health and my life in one or two hours a day. I can't work if I don't have my health."—*Badi SW, NFE class, Nepalgung*

"We thought running NFE classes for the Badi women would be easy. In the beginning, there was full attendance. But slowly, they found that they have got to work hard. Also, the mother would come in saying, 'Daughter, your client is waiting. Hurry and come.' She does not want to lose 50 to 100 Rs, and she'll go.

"Rather than start with adult sex workers, it may be most effective to conduct an out of school program. Badi parents support OSP and want it for their children. The children aren't earning money. Also, the houses are small, so it is good if there is somewhere else for children to go. Maybe we cannot change the behavior of those who are already in that population. But we may change the behavior of those who are small now. The students in our two OSP classes are very good. Soon we will integrate them into school."—*ICH*

"Literacy among the Badi is maybe 8 percent. They would drop out of school because teachers and kids would embarrass them. They had no self-confidence and could not imagine how their own children would go to school. In 1989 with a grant from a Danish NGO we started a hostel/school—not for Badi only, because that would lead to stigmatization. We started with one class and now there are five with 109 students, half girls and half boys. Forty-nine graduates have integrated into government schools. The parents are very much involved, and other districts are asking for the same scheme. Only four girls in four years have been taken back by their mothers to work."—*SAFE*

"MANK works with girls to create HIV/AIDS awareness and educate them about trafficking so they will not end up as sex workers. To stop trafficking we have to address all the social reasons behind it, and one is that girls are kept ignorant. NFE is a place to change that. We don't say, this class will be about HIV/AIDS and girl trafficking. No one would come. We integrate that information later on and tell how a girl who is trafficked unwillingly may be beaten, drugged and raped, how anyone might get HIV in the brothels and bring it back. These are things no one ever talks about, even returned girls. Many girls are terrified to hear this, and some people realize they were selling their girls without knowing what would happen. They say they will try to keep their girls home and convince others. But some just feel this is a normal thing, a tradition. Reactions vary, but the main thing is to make the information available, to talk, read and write about what is concealed.

NFE class alone will not prevent trafficking. But for the girl, there will be a little bit of a change of attitude because she knows how to read and write, knows what happens in a brothel and something about HIV. Maybe she is a little less vulnerable when a boy comes to town and says he has a job for her in the city. However, the Tamang people here have a tradition of love marriages. This is rare in Nepal, but dangerous for the girls, because traffickers can fool them into falling in love, marrying and leaving the village. We can't prevent this, all we can say is check the boy's background. Still, what drives this problem is extreme poverty. Girls are sold to get the money. Girls go to India themselves for the money. They want a better life.

Whether literacy leads to jobs, well, that depends on the person. One girl from the advanced class is now a nurse. But as part of our whole program, it contributes to success. In one ward here every house had trafficked someone in the past, but last year, not one girl went from there."—*MANK*

INCOME GENERATION: Providing alternate income sources for sex workers, potential sex workers and their families is seen as a key component in reducing vulnerability. NGOs have found, however, that they must accept the reality that no alternative can provide the same level of income as sex work. However, alternative incomes may help women limit their partners or refuse partners who will not use condoms. In addition, this kind of intervention is accepted by the general community because it counters the NGOs' image as "promoters" of prostitution because they support sex workers.

"A client fell in love with me and now we are living together as man and wife. Now I'm not doing business any more. SAFE gave my parents a loan for goats, and that money they make from goats is enough to make up for what I gave them. It adds enough to what they get from fishing and such."—*Badi woman, Nepalgung*

"Before, I depended on my two sisters for support. They worked as sex workers. I had a job in construction, but the contract ended. Once, I had my own shop, but I gave too much credit and than some of my family got sick. I got 5,000 Rs from SAFE to open this shop. There is no interest. I agreed to pay back 1000 Rs each year. I put aside 10 Rs a day and paid the first installment early. In my family now, no one is doing the sex business and I am independent. This shop makes enough to support me and my wife and baby daughter. But even if I was not running this shop, I wouldn't send anyone to sex work. I'd get another job. I hate that business. It is socially unaccepted, and so our community has been dominated and exploited." —*Badi shopkeeper, Nepalgung*

"We have a sewing training center for the Badi sex workers and a program to provide support for their families. We don't expect either program to give enough income for total support. But by supplementing the sex workers' income and the family's income, we hope to reduce the number of partners the girls need to have to support the family. That way, she is not compelled to accept clients who refuse to use a condom. Of the fifteen grantees so far, three have already started to pay us back. We feel that the grantee's daughters and sisters truly have found relief. Five sex workers have only one partner now because of this support.

The sewing center is training 22 Badi women now. The Badi chose to learn those skills, and SAFE thought this could introduce alternatives to sex work, and maybe they could move into full time sewing later on. So far, no one has expressed a desire to do that. If they open a tailoring collective they might earn enough to live on, but we can't say that they would be able to save anything." —*SAFE*

"We conduct sewing training and beautician training for the Badi women, but for now, we cannot call them income generating programs. Compared to the sex business, there is little income. At first, we thought they would change the profession. Now we think no, but she might have less partners. Now, we are thinking that we have to broaden our focus to include all the Badi community. Badi men say to us, 'Sir, you are always coming here and talking to our daughters and missing us. Why don't you support us? If we could earn more money, the daughters may not do that business.' They are very interested in taking training for a profession and mention carpentry, wiring or plumbing."—*ICH*

"We have given 30 women a loan to start a business—both sex workers and low caste women who may go to sex work if they don't get support. So far our experience is not too successful. The women are much too poor to repay the loans. One will get a pig, but before it can have babies, she will sell it to buy necessities, then go back to sex work. Our goal is just to support them, give them an alternative, not make them quit their profession. Our activities can be considered as a 'harm reduction project.' It will enable sex workers to increase their self confidence and therefore their power to negotiate safer sex with their clients and perhaps reduce the number of clients they see."—*NESCORD*

LEADERSHIP DEVELOPMENT AND EMPOWERMENT: SAFE and BASE have been able to work with sex workers in this area because the Badi are a cohesive and self-identified group. This makes them an easier target for discrimination, but also easier to organize on their own behalf as a community.

"Before working on HIV with the Badi, SAFE was already responding to pressure against them by authorities by focusing on empowering them for self-help. For example, once the whole town decided to isolate the Badis and blocked their access. The police came and beat the clients and threatened the women. This lasted over a month in 1988. We tried to convince the police that resolving prostitution is a gradual problem and to support their children, sex work is still needed. They did not respond and many families had to sell some assets. Finally, the Badi community united and the youths stood by each house all night. The police stopped the harassment and we could negotiate more. This gave people a taste for their ability to deal with their own problems, it built self-confidence. It also began what is a very slow process of building understanding and easing police pressure."—*SAFE*

A SAFER FUTURE FOR SEX WORKERS AND THEIR CLIENTS

Little information is available about what, in the context of Nepal, determines a decision to purchase sex, and research on this might lead to interventions that would help clients better understand, and thus change, their behavior. This knowledge might also contribute to developing interventions that could help sex workers negotiate on their own behalf with clients, pimps or hotel/brothel owners, family and authorities.

Outreach to sex workers is difficult and time consuming and there are very large sex worker populations that have not yet been targeted, particularly in the Kathmandu Valley. Research to develop outreach techniques could be valuable, and appropriate interventions might include a range of programs from expanded STD detection and referral to clinics that provide HIV/AIDS education to advocacy for sex workers' rights and decriminalization of commercial sex. For sex workers with whom contact has been made, one area of research might be on developing their skills in negotiating condom use with clients and other partners.

The difficulties involved in outreach to sex workers returning from high prevalence areas also pose questions: Should voluntary HIV testing be recommended? How could counseling and support services be created to reach this invisible population? What alternate income generation would be effective for sex workers with HIV/AIDS? What support systems would be appropriate?

Economic forces, stigmatization and pressure from authorities can lead sex workers to hide or not to investigate their health status. This has both health and human rights ramifications that raise serious questions for the future. For example, because sex workers are a population often chosen for the purpose of HIV surveillance through systematic blood testing, their rights to privacy and confidentiality are vulnerable. SAFE, for one, is concerned about developing policy on blood testing: "Many organizations want to test Badi sex workers' blood and our dilemma is whether to recommend that they allow it. We counseled the Badi in Rajapur recently not to give blood until the group asking for it contacted SAFE, because all of the women weren't aware of confidentiality and what blood testing can imply. The group didn't do the test or contact us. In Nepalgung, they have decided not to give blood for testing any more. After all, if one of the girls turns out to have HIV, what will happen to her? We feel we would have to be responsive to the government if they wanted to do a study and would guarantee anonymity, but it would be a hard decision that would involve the Badi, the people in our network, the NGOs, and our international funders."

The need for developing this kind of multi-level approach is also stressed by MANK and WOREC as the only way to stop trafficking. It would require interventions coordinating rights advocacy for young girls and women, economic development and government cooperation.

THE BADI COMMUNITY

The Badi are the lowest ranking untouchable caste in far western Nepal where they live. Badi men have no traditional service. The Badi are thought to have come from India in the 14th century as traveling singers, dancers, and storytellers. (In the Hindu belief system, untouchable groups are each matched to specific services and the Badi are matched to entertainment.) Wealthy Nepali patrons provided them with land and filled basic needs in return for entertainment and sex. After 1950, when political reforms diminished the patrons' wealth, Badi women turned increasingly to sex work, which was in greater demand as the population in their area grew.

Badi children understand that females of their caste support their families with sex work, which begins soon after first menstruation. A woman usually leaves the profession when her daughters can earn enough to support her, or if she marries or grows too old. Working sex workers earn between 3,000 and 7,000 Rs a month. Few Badi women marry, though in a family with three or four daughters working, additional daughters may be free to do so. The Badi travel frequently among Badi towns, and a broad network of community support and interaction exists.

[Adapted in part from 'The Badi: Prostitution as a Social Norm Among an Untouchable Cast of West Nepal' by Thomas Cox, in *Quarterly Development Review*, Vol. X, #13.]

INCREASING SEX WORKERS' LITERACY

Twenty women between the ages of 16 and 39, a few holding infants, sit on the floor of a small second-story room in Nepalgung. The temperature is over 110 degrees and the facilitator must also compete with extremely loud music from the street. These women are less shy and far more likely to have an opinion and voice it than most Nepali women I've encountered. Their individual personalities seem apparent even on first meeting, and I wonder if this stronger sense of self is tied to the fact that they are valued from birth as potential wage earners—as boys are elsewhere in the society. I ask them what they have learned here and whether being literate will change anything for them:

"Now I can tell people I've been to NFE and I know more. It is important to be able to say 'I am literate.'"

"When I became a sex worker, I didn't know anything about the world outside. Now, I know through this class that sex work is a bad thing. I won't let my daughters do this. If I can get a good education for my children, they can find another type of work and I can be supported by them."

"Even if I get very good training, I never expect to join a bank or an INGO or some big business. Even if we did, we'd be recognized as Badi and it would be expected that we would give sex. It's better that we concentrate on small things, like running a tea stall or shop to get income, and to do that, you need to read and know numbers."

Although some of the women seem eager to talk, others continue to work quietly in their books, and a few slip out before class is over. Given my intrusion, they may feel that the time would be better spent working.

"I worked at different places in Delhi for eight years and came home every year for major festivals. I had heard the word HIV in India, but I never heard any details before I saw the presentation today. I'm not worried about HIV, but now I know a person should be safe all the time. Then you don't have to worry, do you?"—MIGRANT FACTORY WORKER, POKHARA

CHAPTER 6

WHEN THE TARGET IS ALWAYS ON THE MOVE: NEPAL'S MOBILE WORKERS

While some 90 percent of Nepal's population is reported to be rural and agriculturally based, much of it is also surprisingly mobile. This mobility is being facilitated by Nepal's growing network of roads and highways connecting urban centers with each other and with India. Each year, some 800,000 Nepalis migrate to India to work and two million or more Indian truck drivers, farm workers and sellers enter Nepal.

One large mobile population, migrants who work in Nepal's factories, is discussed in *Chapter 7*. Others, discussed here, include migrant workers outside factories, transportation workers, and members of the police and military forces who are stationed away from home. Despite broad differences in what makes them vulnerable to HIV, these groups have much in common: All are far from home, family and their locus of common values for long periods of time. They share common risk factors, the most usual being having multiple sexual partners (sex workers, "second wives" and/or homosexual contacts). They also may put their partners at risk when they return home, and they set a common challenge for the NGOs because their mobility makes outreach and follow-up difficult.

TRANSPORT WORKERS

This almost exclusively male group includes bus and truck drivers and their helpers. Truck drivers, in particular, enjoy considerable prestige in both Nepal and India and earn high salaries supplemented by independent hauling contracts. In a country where most transportation is still by foot, a man with a truck is king. Drivers are seen as being sophisticated, widely traveled and full of sexual prowess. An unknown but high percentage of truck drivers patronize sex workers at stops along the major highways and at their final destinations. A NESCORD survey found that 55 percent to 64 percent of long-distance drivers reported visiting sex workers while away from home. There is a belief that "heat" generated after long drives needs to be cooled off by ejaculation and that condoms act as a barrier to releasing this heat. If no sex worker is available, some drivers may have anal sex with their helpers, who cannot object because they are in the position of a pupil to a guru. Many truck drivers are aware that HIV has spread along trucking routes in Africa and are sensitive to being stigmatized for bringing AIDS from India to Nepal.

Bus drivers' risk behavior may be similar to truckers', but they are on tighter schedules and have less opportunity to stop enroute. The category of helpers can include employees such as bus conductors, apprentice drivers who serve as general help, and low-paid, transient laborers.

Risk reduction interventions targeting transport workers have focused on providing IEC, condoms and STD referral. Access to these men is difficult because they are rarely at home and have little time while on the road to sit for HIV/AIDS education or attend workshops. Interpersonal communications have been found effective. Behavior change counseling is available from the NGOs targeting this population, but it is not yet well developed and few from the target population have taken advantage of it. One NGO makes education and counseling available to truckers' wives as well, but this focus may become a source of family friction.

"At first, we set up educational seminars and group discussions in town, but the drivers were reluctant to attend. And we were only approaching the drivers, which made them ask, 'Why only us? Why do you always talk about truck drivers?' So now we say 'transport workers.' Later, we decided to reach them by showing a video with an AIDS message at the bus park. We also gave out cassette tapes of popular music with AIDS messages in between. Then they started coming up with questions. They also said they wanted information, free condoms and more educational materials available in the bus park, so we set up a booth. But it has still been difficult. The man in charge at the booth was not from the community, and that might have been a problem. The service is still more education than counseling, but now when I go there, the men make a point to show me that they have condoms with them."—*ICH*

"Before we began AIDS education at the bus park, we discussed it with the transport association. They agreed that the workers are at risk and they provided a place for the booth. In the first three months, there were 444 visitors. At first, the drivers thought we were targeting only them, but we convinced them by saying the bus park is a public place where a lot of people can get our information.

"Our sign says 'AIDS Education and Prevention' and that brings people over. What they want to know about most is sexuality and the diseases it causes. Where else can they ask these questions? Some even tell about their sexual behavior with their wife, or ask questions like, 'When I can't get erect with a condom is the lubrication doing something to me?' Seven men have come specifically for advice and referral about their STD—we thought there would be more. People also want posters and pamphlets to take to their village.

"We expected follow up questions, but only three or four men have come back. There is a huge turn-over here. Assistants can have a fight with the driver and never show up again. We don't know if they get enough information in one visit to change their behavior. We do know they take condoms."—*SAFE*

"In our target area there are some 1700 transport drivers and their families, but it is very hard to reach them. We tried to recruit drivers to be in our peer educator group. Some former drivers joined, but no one who is working now. So we thought to bring the education to them through their wives. At first it was very difficult to make it clear we were not accusing their husbands of anything, that we were bringing information only. We tell the wives they can make sure their husbands use a condom with them, because they can't know what the men do outside."—*NESCORD*

THE POLICE AND MILITARY FORCES

"Those boys [police] can create a lot of disturbance. They come and harass us and the clients. We had five clients who came from India and the cops came here when they were leaving and took all their money and chased them away. Sometimes they have tried to rape us. We have gone to SAFE with these problems."— *Badi CSW in Nepalgung*

The police and military forces are predominantly male, although there are some policewomen. They live in barracks and can be stationed away from home for one to three years at a time. They are government workers with some education but are not highly paid. Members of these services wield considerable power, but the police in particular are not highly respected. Both groups are often ignorant about their risks for HIV that include patronizing sex workers and the male to male sex that reportedly takes place in the barracks. Some UN soldiers reportedly don't know which countries have a high prevalence of HIV, and they do not receive education on HIV before being transferred abroad. There is an urgent need to educate members of both the police and military on HIV/AIDS, and several AmFAR partner NGOs have already begun to do so.

These populations need HIV education not only with respect to their own personal behavior, but also so that they can understand the life circumstances and HIV risks of populations under their jurisdiction. Some of the NGOs targeting police approach them as an independent, at-risk population. Others, particularly NGOs working with sex workers and IDUs, educate the police because it also benefits their primary target. Perhaps because of their education level, NGOs have found that the HIV message is readily understood by these groups. Follow-up can be difficult because of frequent transfers, and little counseling for behavior change has been initiated. Some police groups have already incorporated an HIV/AIDS component into the drug awareness program they present at schools.

"One sex worker mentioned that the police are not interested in using condoms and said if we could train them, that would be helpful. So we conducted two one-day sessions for local police and their supervisors. Our post-test showed that after one session, they are aware about AIDS. Now they see that AIDS information is important for them, also. This also established some good relations. There is still harassment of the sex workers, but less than before. Education helps, but a community has to find its own solution. We can assist them only.

"It is not a problem we can solve on this level. Police are in power and they misuse that power. Our plan is to expand the program through the network as much as possible with our resources. If we educate the policemen from this area, some of them will coordinate with other people. Also, we often involve interested people from other areas in our trainings so they can do a program at home. This can be a possibility for educating the police also."—*SAFE*

THE GURKHA

"We got started in AIDS education through our theater group. Before, the old men thought it was just rubbish to make noise and bring crowds. But now we go around performing the AIDS street drama, and the old men think we are doing something really good for our community."
—*WICOM AIDS educator, Sainik Basti*

Traditionally drawn from among four of Nepal's Tibeto-Burman groups (Magars, Gurungs, Rais and Limbus), members of the Ghurkha regiments now come from nearly every ethnic group, though Tibeto-Burmans predominate heavily. The Ghurkhas serve in foreign armies abroad and return home for a few months every two or three years. Their foreign earnings make their families and villages enormously prosperous by Nepal's standards. Ghurkha soldiers abroad, particularly those in the British army, have access to health care and information and education on HIV/AIDS and STDs, yet STD rates among Ghurkha couples in Nepal is reported to be high. Ghurkha's wives may be at risk for HIV from their returning husbands, and may also have other sexual partners during the long periods of separation. WICOM targets the 300 Ghurkha families living in Sainik Basti near Pokhara.

"This group is economically more sophisticated than most Nepalis, but with respect to sex education—no. The first year we brought the community together for mass education, but they would not come a second time. Most of the women work at home spinning or in the fields and don't think it is appropriate to go out for such information. The youth were more enthusiastic, so we began HIV education in the schools, but students were not taking the information home. So now we have an intra-family strategy and do house to house visits. We two educators are from that community and often related. The women welcome us into their home, and are not embarrassed to discuss these matters with us. People say it is something they should know because AIDS could be an epidemic in the future. But WICOM has had no success with teaching the women condom negotiation. For example, one woman tried to talk to her husband who had returned from Korea and he said, 'There is no AIDS in Korea!' The counselor had tried to tell her, 'Use a condom until you are sure he hasn't been unfaithful. Until he opens up and is honest.' But not one woman had been successful."—*WICOM*

MIGRANT LABORERS

"The Danuwar community is very discriminated against. They live surrounded by hills that keep them isolated from other communities and they are afraid of external influence. So when they go for work, they want to go outside Nepal, they go to India."—*DSS*

The decision to migrate in search of employment is most often driven by economic necessity in Nepal, although, especially for some young people, the mystique of urban life may also beckon. Most migration is within Nepal and between Nepal and India, although Nepali laborers also go to other countries. The 1991 census shows that nearly 4 percent of the population migrates seasonally to India. MANK reports that 25 percent of the young people from the area they serve migrates to India. Before 1992, the majority of migrants were males, but an increasing number of females now go as well, often accompanying their husbands. These migrant women usually work in factories or as manual labor on construction and road building projects in Nepal and India. Some migrants work away from home only during the six months a year when fields are fallow. Others find longer-term jobs and return home periodically, usually for religious festivals. Migrant men patronize sex workers and may have a "second wife." Wives left at home may take other partners. STD rates among migrant workers are reportedly high. Unlike the "career" migrants discussed above, migrant laborers are additionally vulnerable because of social and economic factors such as poverty, lack of access to services, illiteracy, and caste or ethnic discrimination.

Interventions targeting this population have focused on outreach and providing IEC and condoms. Follow-up and behavior change interventions have not been implemented. However, many migrants and would-be migrants are among the target populations of several NGOs that offer programs in their villages such as NFE classes with HIV/AIDS components.

"It is our experience as physicians that young migrant men have many STDs when they come home. In deciding how to approach them, we found out which routes they use to go to India and found two crossings used by migrants from six districts in the surrounding hills. We have peer educators there to give information, education and free condoms. But we found they are not necessarily going to stop for us. So we approach the ones who stop at the customs house and ask them to respond to our questionnaire that introduces the topic of HIV/AIDS. After they answer the questions, it is easier to talk more with them."—*ICH*

"Maybe 1000 Danuwar go to India each year from this district. We try to get HIV education to them before they leave home. AIDS education is given through mass meetings and our field workers also visit homes door to door. It is a very hard task, especially to educate people to practice condom use. It is not possible to follow up this education, because they go away. Even though we are from the Danuwar community, we have found resistance to our program. One problem is tradition. They are afraid of any external influence and they won't mention their problems to others. They stay with their own traditions, their own festivals and culture."—*DSS*

FUTURE INTERVENTIONS
FOR MOBILE POPULATIONS

Because mobility so limits access to these communities, it may be important to develop additional strategies to improve that access, perhaps by researching catchment areas and sub-population-specific approaches. Involving peers may be one approach to the problem of follow-up and counseling for behavior change, but almost nothing is known about what determines the sexual behavior of these groups, and this kind of research may be necessary to establish effective interventions.

One important but very difficult question is what can reasonably be advised to both men and women in the case of returned migrant laborers. Should they, for example, rely on visible evidence of an STD? Is it realistic to tell women they must use condoms if they can assume their husband had contact with sex workers? For how long? A related question is what role voluntary HIV testing might play for returning migrants. There is no clear answer, and strategies and guidelines need to be researched.

Coordination with the government could be valuable in bringing HIV/AIDS education to the police and military. It might be possible, for example, to arrange for the education to become part of basic training and to include training that would develop peer educators within each class. Another area for coordination with the government may be challenging the misuse of power by these groups. ICH frames the problem in terms of resolving the tension between the law and the sex workers' livelihood: "This profession is not legal and the police are duty bound to honor this. At the same time, they should not harass the sex workers in extreme ways—like by spreading rumors that they have HIV. It could drive some of them mad, and it destroys the entire community. This creates problems that really have to be solved on the national level."

CHAPTER 7

WORKING TOGETHER EVERY DAY: MEN AND WOMEN IN NEPAL'S FACTORIES

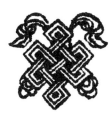Relatively large numbers of people at risk for and vulnerable to HIV gather in Nepal's factories six days a week. In Nepal manufacturing that is on a larger scale than village handicrafts clusters around urban centers and produces a wide variety of domestic consumer goods from batteries to soft drinks to cement. Carpet factories produce 60 percent of Nepal's export income. Most factories are small and much—in some cases all—of the work is done by hand. This sector of the economy is fueled by an increasing number of men, women and children looking for work in urban centers. The majority of factory workers today are young adults, as child labor

laws have been more strictly enforced in the past year. (HIV/AIDS education for children working in factories is discussed in *Chapter 4*.) Some factories have powerful unions and a fairly stable, salaried labor force working regular hours. In others, notably carpet factories, worker turnover is high, earnings are lower and payment is by the piece. Generally, women, children and carpet factory workers earn less than men and union workers.

RISK BEHAVIORS AND FACTORS INFLUENCING RISK

Many factory employees are migrant workers. They move among factories and between where they work and their home village. Factory settings have gotten a reputation for prostitution and sexual exploitation of female workers, but it has not been documented. Workers' risk of exposure to multiple partners is nevertheless high. As one worker observed, "People get attracted." Women, who earn less, may turn to occasional sex work to supplement their incomes or may be pressured to give or sell sex by men with jurisdiction over them. Access to condoms is likely to be better than in villages, but condom use remains low. STD rates are unknown, but are presumed by NGOs to be relatively high. NGOs with programs in factories stress the need for general health care on site.

HIV PREVENTION IN THE WORKPLACE

"My problem is, I can't give classes as often as I want because I need permission from management. I would do AIDS education all the time if I could."—*Bharav Phatak, WICOM factory peer educator, Kathmandu.*

AmFAR partner NGOs have designed HIV/AIDS programs for factories in many areas of Nepal. They report that factory workers in the greater Kathmandu area generally show less interest in HIV/AIDS information than workers in more rural settings. Risk reduction interventions used in the factories have included IEC, condom promotion and distribution, counseling and provision of basic health care.

GAINING ACCESS: Every NGO targeting factory workers encountered initial resistance from owners and winning their support was a struggle. After two years, some owners and managers still show resistance, but others are supportive and some are considering contributing funds to the programs. In factories with unions, gaining the leaders' cooperation proved crucial. The NGOs found that the situation in carpet factories was not analogous to that in other types of factory.

"Management was afraid we were investigating childrens' working conditions, so they were resistant. It took two or three months of personal contacts, meetings with the carpet association and so on to convince the majority of them. Also, we formed a committee of factory owners' wives that was very useful. Management saw that it would benefit from our program, too. For example, we offered general health care and referrals for workers. That meant the factory can advertise: 'We have health and education facilities,' and this impresses the international market, especially Europe. Also, carpet workers get paid by the square meter and can work any hours, so managers can't object that our program cuts productivity.

"If we only did education in the factory, we couldn't really cover the target population. Migration can make it hard to know who has gotten our classes. So it is important that workers have access to us inside and outside the factory. We try to encourage them to come to our center by offering videos, street drama, HIV and general health counseling there."—*CDS*

"We had to use personal connections and meetings with the owners to gain acceptance. They were concerned that we would interrupt production, and most of their workers are on salary. But these people do not live on site and we wanted to reach them during working hours because family responsibilities and transportation problems can make staying after work difficult. Our program takes two hours, but management was most reluctant to allow more than one. We encouraged them to observe our education and street drama, and that gained support for expanding to two hours. A significant achievement is that this year management personnel often participate in our education sessions.

"The political change in Nepal has strengthened the workers unions and now organizing our programs must include meetings with union leaders to get their agreement. Where the union is of the Marxist-Leninist party, they seem to be against NGOs for political reasons, so there may be resistance. It is not easy to get into the factories unless you have regular, informal meetings with many people—managers, unions, political leaders, social workers, elders—and involve them and get their participation if possible."—*WICOM*

IEC: Once inside the factories, the NGOs often found that the populations were more diverse than they had anticipated and their needs did not correspond to pre-conceived ideas. During year one, this often meant making changes in how the HIV education was presented.

"Before I started being a peer educator, I had the idea that HIV/AIDS was trivial...a sex workers disease. When I talk about AIDS in the factory, people listen so well it really inspires me. I get the feeling their attitudes have changed after attending the class. They ask me questions and they completely understand that this disease is fatal. I realize I have a big responsibility to see that people get the *right* message."—*Pharav Phatak, WICOM factory peer educator, Kathmandu*

"Some of my co-workers say that AIDS education in the factory is important because it is exclusively for them and gives details—not like a short message on the radio. They are also glad it comes to them. People are so busy in their life, I don't think they would go looking somewhere else for AIDS education."
—*Lal Singh Tamang, WICOM factory peer educator, Pokhara*

"Even if you are in the field every day, it takes time to learn about your target population. It took us over six months to see the details of the factory structure. For example, we learned that in addition to weavers, we also had to target the washers and dyers, who often speak only the Maithali language, so it was more difficult than we thought. At first, we talked to workers one-on-one. This was very time consuming, so we changed to groups. We started with men and women together, but the women did not participate, so we separated them. These groups were held in the open, which was very distracting, so we negotiated with managers to provide a room. Now things are more efficient.

"We have had success with peer educators in several factories. Most are campus students, so they are different from the target population but still peers in that they work inside the factory. We chose people who are really interested and gave them six trainings. They do HIV/AIDS education in their factory and also save us a lot of time by scheduling our educations with management and making sure everyone is present on time. They also promote health messages, like using face masks, to workers and management. We have found that you have to hammer away at the message all the time. You cannot stop or take it for granted that *any* population has been covered and will change their behavior. We go to each factory once a week, if we skip a week or there's a month's holiday, they forget. Every week—forever maybe. But if you go often, you can't bore them with the same material. So one week, we do a flip chart then next time we ask, 'How did you like the flip chart?' The next week, street drama. Then, 'How did you like the street drama?' Everyone likes the street dramas. People pay attention to what is entertaining, and there is not much of that in AIDS education.

"We think workers are getting the message. What they say shows more understanding now. For example, married women didn't ask anything about mother to child transmission at first, even though it was explained on the flip chart. After a year, they are saying, 'I don't know about my husband, maybe I am positive, what about my baby?' We explain from the first that many HIV positive married women only had contact with their husband. The women discuss this and decide, 'Oh, it must be from the husband!' But it takes a long time before they think, 'Maybe *my* husband, too!'"—*CDS*

"At first we did education with males and females together, but the workers and the peer educators said it made people too shy because it discusses condoms and sex. Having separate sessions has improved female participation, but not to the level of men. It can take six or seven sessions for people to open up and start asking questions openly in meetings. We were using pre- and post-tests to measure how well people understood the education, but that was especially difficult because most workers are illiterate and explaining took time away from the presentation and the follow-up questions. Now we do random interviews after the street drama and hold a small focus group after the education session. We have 36 peer educators in the factories, and one problem we find is that sometimes they aren't given time off to do educations, and when they do get released, the other workers wonder why."—*WICOM*

CONDOM PROMOTION AND DISTRIBUTION: All the NGOs targeting factories promote, demonstrate and distribute condoms. Condoms are made available at the factory from peer educators and/or conveniently placed boxes. One NGO distributes them at a nearby tea shop. They are also available at the NGOs' offices. It has been especially difficult, particularly in carpet factories, to convince women to take condoms.

"The factory atmosphere combines both sexes. People get attracted. Married and unmarried men have asked me for a condom. Once after a presentation many women asked me for condoms. But they were all married, so they could do that openly."—*Lal Singh Tamang, WICOM peer educator, Pokhara*

"I'm married and have two children and I am using condoms now. If we had alternative family planning, maybe I wouldn't use condoms. You feel more safe from pregnancy with the other, but when you think of HIV... I sometimes take condoms and pamphlets from here as a present to other factory workers. I tell my friends back home about this, too. They used to think they could get HIV from a sneeze or a toilet. I tell them, 'You should know about this, if you make a little mistake, you've had it.'"—*Min Bahadur, 20, carpet weaver, Kathmandu*

"We had trouble introducing condoms. Most of the adult carpet workers were married, and they had seen condoms from family planning workers who stressed sterilization as more reliable. At first, we also provided those, but we learned that other family planning methods interfere with condom use. Women especially have trouble with the idea of insisting on a condom if they are on another form of birth control. And men with vasectomies ask, 'How will I face my wife?' After a year and a half the women are still very shy about talking with us about condom use or being seen taking condoms. Having peer educators in the factory helps because they can talk to someone of their own sex in confidence.

"So at first no one took the condoms seriously. We put out a box and it would disappear. They would blow them up, management complained condoms were blocking the toilets. We said, well, at least people know what condoms look like now. Slowly it changed. Wastage has stopped and we think that is a good indicator. People take as many as 200 a week from some boxes. We got condoms accepted by constantly saying, 'It's not only for family planning, it is for STDs and AIDS.' Stressing this

makes them take condoms more seriously because most of them have STDs. Now we are trying to motivate people to buy condoms when they need them, not just wait and get them free from us. We feel that people will use condoms only as long as we provide them free, but for how long can we continue to do that?"
—*CDS*

HEALTH CARE: few factories provide on-site clinics, but for most workers, access to health care is difficult and there is a tendency to wait until problems are acute before seeking treatment. In its second project year, NCWCA brought limited health care to non-carpet factories in Bhaktapur and encountered the same problems that caused CDS to cut back its first year health care program—insufficient budget to meet the very high demand for medications.

"CDS began as an NGO with a clinic. At the beginning, that made it easier to introduce the topic of HIV—to be able to say, 'We've come not only to talk about AIDS but about hygiene, sanitation and so on.' People know what to expect from us now and we don't have to approach the topic so carefully any more. When we wrote the AmFAR project proposal, I was working in the county hospital and women from the carpet factory would come with children who were very undernourished and in the last stages of diseases like meningitis. One of the mothers was HIV positive. It seemed important to make some health care available inside the factories, to catch things sooner. But now we have moved to more general health counseling. We started a referral clinic last year as one way to attract women to come to our office. And they did come. The decision to move away from providing care was partly due to a lack of a regular supply of the medications to treat more and more clients from the factories."—*CDS*

INFORMING AND EDUCATING THE WORK FORCE

The NGOs have approached factory workers with targeted IEC, condom promotion and distribution, and STD referral in the context of general health care and counseling. But these do not address the context of workers' lives which makes the "constant hammering away" necessary. The foundation of much of their vulnerability is the context of migration, which is discussed in detail in Chapter 6. Another factor is illiteracy, which makes comprehending even basic health messages more difficult. Females, who are paid less and often have children to care for and household duties in addition to their employment, are especially vulnerable to sexual exploitation (for money or to keep their job). Competition for jobs is high and increasing, giving workers less bargaining power to negotiate for basic rights and better pay and working conditions.

The NGOs' interventions to reduce vulnerability for this population have focused primarily on providing NFE classes with an HIV/AIDS component. Steps are also beginning to be taken toward establishing alternative income generation opportunities in the villages and organizing lobbying for better working conditions. Both CDS and NCWCA have provided NFE classes for carpet factory workers. NCWCA found that women in Bhaktapur factories wanted to learn basic English and math in addition to basic literacy because they felt that those skills would improve their chances of employment at trekking sites near their home villages. NCWCA now works in non-carpet factories and has offered to train facilitators if management takes responsibility for providing NFE. Whether they will do so, and whether NFE is a good approach in that setting remains to be seen.

"I get up at six and go to work until nine. Then I go home to cook breakfast and eat with my family. At eleven I come to NFE for two hours. Then I go to weave until seven when I go home for tea. I go back and weave until eleven then go home and eat supper. My father cooks it because my mother went back to the village recently. I wanted to come to NFE because I didn't understand the alphabet or how to count. Also, I didn't understand anything about HIV or about health. Now this class is catching me up. Maybe if I can study, I can get a job. Most of all, I'd like to go back to my village and teach."—*Thuli Maya, 19, carpet weaver, Kathmandu*

"We conduct ten NFE classes of 30 students each, some are for children. About 60 percent of the students are male, 40 percent female, and 35 percent to 50 percent will drop out eventually. But those who stay come consistently. Two women who now work six kilometers away come here by three-wheel taxis every day. The women who come to NFE often have very specific reasons. The two most common are that they want the privacy of being able to read for themselves the letters they receive, and they want to be able to understand their receipts so they are not cheated. When they first come, they just want to study, study, study. They are only interested in learning letters and numbers. We found that if we put in the HIV/AIDS element right away, they just say, 'Oh, this is going to be the same thing we get in the factory,' and they drop out. So we wait about two months until they have enough basics to follow it in the book. A lot of these women think carpet work is only temporary and if they can read, they can get a better job. That will be hard, but literacy can make a difference."—*CDS*

IMPROVING WORKERS' QUALITY OF LIFE

Organizations working in factories are beginning to see a broader spectrum of sub-populations than they originally had targeted. Research to design interventions appropriate for owners, managers, clerical staff, union leaders and supervisors might be considered, especially given the influence these groups can have on workplace conditions.

One approach to reducing the vulnerability of migrant factory workers might be to consider ways to bolster the rural economy so that migration is reduced. CDS is lobbying for a comprehensive approach to the problem. "We have suggested to the government and NGOs that they start income generating projects in the villages, small projects throughout the country—like producing wool for the carpets. This approach was successful in Thailand where there was also a serious migration and child labor problem in Bangkok. We have sent many letters to the Nepal government and even talked to the Prime Minister and then the Vice Chairman of the planning commission. They said, 'Oh, that's a good idea, we will think about it.' We have heard nothing yet." Examining the Thai model for lessons relevant to Nepal could be valuable for future interventions. Skill training and alternate income generation for carpet factory workers might also be considered, especially as many of them already consider carpet work a temporary step to something better.

Improvements in the working environment and in workers' quality of life may decrease their vulnerability to HIV. More investigation is needed to see who can best provide either on-site education, housing, health care and child care, or improved off-site access to these.

AT THE MAHU GURU CARPET FACTORY

One enters this small Kathmandu carpet factory through a narrow door in a brick wall that opens onto a courtyard flanked by several small buildings. The weaving area is bright and airy and sports electric blue loom frames. The small room for NFE classes is close, hot and windowless. It is very quiet, not only because everything is done by hand here, but also because when I arrive, everyone is watching a CDS street drama in the courtyard. The owner, Raju Lama, is happily taking photos, but breaks off to tell me how enthusiastic he is about the HIV/AIDS program.

"The workers should get this knowledge. Before, they didn't even know what sex is, how to survive in the city. Now, they are more free and open, less frightened of life. It's like they are beginning to know who they are.

"When CDS first came, I asked around and decided they were OK. I am a factory owner now, but I also have had to struggle in life. I thought, if these workers get an opportunity, they can do something with themselves. I put myself in their place. I tell other owners about this program and promote it. Some agree and some say, why waste the working time? To them I say, 'Because of you, 50 people will suffer from lack of knowledge about HIV, from a lack of other education. Why deprive them?'"

HIV/AIDS EDUCATION AT A POULTRY FEED FACTORY

It's 3 PM, and this Kathmandu poultry feed factory has closed two hours early. Three groups of men wait in a large, bare room for the HIV/AIDS education to start: Three managers, wearing white shirts and ties, sit on chairs along the wall; six staff members, in casual western clothes, sit on benches in the middle; and a dozen workers cluster on the floor to one side, their ragged T-shirts and shorts powdered with grain dust. Neighborhood men, women and children gather at the windows and doors.

The WICOM staff looks elegant in bright saris and everyone listens intently to the introductory information. After the educator explains modes of transmission, people are urged to participate. The boss cracks a joke and a staff member asks a question. The workers are silent, but attentive, but when the educator urges them to participate they just smile and draw back. Little effort is made to engage them after this.

Condoms are passed around and the workers have to be coaxed to open one and take a look. By the time its proper use is demonstrated on a stylized wooden penis, the windows are packed with onlookers. After half an hour, when the talk turns to STDs, the workers' attention begins to flag, but the others are fully engaged. They ask: "How safe is the blood supply?" "What is homosexuality?" "Why is HIV spreading if you are doing this program?" and "How many girls do I have to go to before I get sick?," which makes everyone laugh.

Afterwards, everyone gathers on a grassy strip separating the factory from a wide, noisy street. The site was chosen to attract passersby to the street drama. The crowd is mostly male, though the age range is wide. Three old women bearing huge bundles of fodder watch from a distance, though they cannot possibly hear. The plot revolves around a village man who has not heard from his son in Kathmandu in months. The man and his grandson decide to go to Kathmandu where their village naiveté is the brunt of much slapstick comedy. They encounter a fellow villager who tells them the son is sick with AIDS. The son enters, followed by an actor representing the HIV virus who gives information about transmission and stresses that AIDS is incurable.

The son says, "It is my karma to die here," and the subject turns to rehabilitation within the community. Misconceptions about HIV are corrected by the various characters, and the son is convinced to return home and become an activist for AIDS education and community understanding. After bows, the troop urges people to stay and ask questions and a few do so, but most quickly head home. It's 5 PM, quitting time.

CHAPTER 8

HARM REDUCTION AND BEHAVIOR CHANGE: INJECTING DRUG USERS

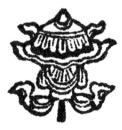 Primarily an urban phenomenon, injecting drug use in Nepal is not well documented. It is, however, highly stigmatized. Estimates of the number of drug users in Nepal range from 25,000 to 40,000, perhaps 10 percent of whom are believed to inject. LALS, the only NGO targeting IDUs, estimates that some 2,000 IDUs reside in its service area, greater Kathmandu. The majority of LALS' clients are men in their 20s, and a large number of them live on the streets and work as casual laborers. Ninety five percent of them were born in Nepal. The population is not homogeneous, however. Needle exchange clients in Kathmandu

range in age from 12 to over 70. About 6 percent are female and 15 percent to 20 percent are street children.

Injecting with a group and needle sharing are common practices in Nepal. Although there are no known equivalents to shooting galleries, groups may gather in known places to inject. As many as 20 individuals have been reported to share a single syringe, though the usual number is much lower. As of October 1995, nine IDUs (8 male, 1 female) had tested positive for HIV. The mode of transmission for all of them is listed as "sexual." Female IDUs may trade sex for drugs or may sell sex for cash to buy drugs. Until recently, brown sugar heroin was the most commonly injected drug. But heroin is becoming more expensive, and people are changing to other drugs. Injecting behavior may be increasing as people switch from inhaling drugs to the more cost effective injecting. About 30 percent of Nepal's IDUs are believed to have traveled to neighboring countries—usually India.

RISK REDUCTION: CONDOMS, CLEAN NEEDLES, AND COUNSELING

LALS has 64 areas where community health outreach workers (CHOWs) make regular contact with IDUs. Risk reduction interventions include needle exchange, provision of bleach and distilled water, some health care, condoms promotion and distribution, and IEC. This is a wary population that migrates following drug sources or because of police pressure, but LALS' program has been very successful, and the current number of needle exchange clients is about 800.

"No one but LALS ever, ever comes here."—*Female IDU/SW living in a vacant lot in Kathmandu*

LALS has the difficult task of having to take an information/education/communication approach not only to its target population, but also to authorities and the general community on an on-going basis. LALS provides awareness raising about drug use and HIV/AIDS to both IDUs and the general public during their field visits. The presentation also includes condom demonstrations and distribution. Many IDUs take condoms and, according to LALS, say they use them. The level of HIV/AIDS awareness among steady clients has increased to the point that they can and do give the presentation themselves.

"Making the first contact and setting up a routine for when and where we will meet is difficult. But once the routine is set, as long as we don't break it, it is easy to make further contacts. One person tells another, and word gets around. The problem is, this population is very mobile and when they move, the counseling and education process breaks. If we find them again, we have to start from the beginning. The main thing we have learned is that without the right attitude and approach, we will not be effective. Because we are working with a population people don't like, may even hate, our policy is to be non-judgmental, non-coercive, and have a respectful, positive attitude. Without this we cannot get their confidence and learn what they need and why they are doing drugs. And without this knowledge, we cannot do effective counseling for behavior change. Another way we learn their needs is to have ex-IDUs on our staff and board.

"Maintaining confidentiality and anonymity are also crucial, but we also have to maintain good relations and constant contact with the authorities, because they could make access very difficult. Sometimes we can have trouble with the police in a new district. They may follow our CHOWs, the community health outreach workers, and maybe intervene in the exchange. Some CHOWs have been arrested briefly. But once we explain exactly why we do the exchange...well, most police people have a heart, and they come to support us. The main thing is, we should always be able to make the authorities and community understand exactly what we are doing in a way that will build support.

"This is a difficult job. People from the general population are always asking us, 'How long did you do drugs?,' asking the women 'Do you have experience as a prostitute?' or accusing us of encouraging drug use. And very occasionally clients can be difficult if they are on certain kinds of drugs. When we recruited our staff we put much more emphasis on their attitude than on their education or experience. So we try to run LALS in an egalitarian way and the structure is participatory."—*LALS*

LALS has had to negotiate at length with the government over the needle exchange program, which the government feels is much too high profile. LALS argues that needle exchange is not illegal because it is an intervention program, and so far the authorities have accepted that. LALS will provide 42,000 needles to 800 IDUs during the program's second year. According to LALS, many of their clients no longer share needles and those who do, share with far fewer people, usually only one or two. Use of bleach and distilled water to sterilize syringes and needles has also increased. The NGO reports that there has been no spread of HIV among their client IDUs.

"I'm surprised this program even exists for us. Before, none of us knew about this, about our risk. We heard all kinds of wrong information about AIDS."—*Male IDU, Kathmandu*

"Needle exchange is not the same thing as creating long term behavior change. The motivations are different. First, a shared needle gets dull and hurts. Second, they want to save money. Last is because they don't want to share with others, and *that* is the point we need to focus on or they will go back to sharing if they are in a hurry or they're sick or whatever. Anything that disrupts the usual routine can lead to sharing if the HIV prevention message has not really taken hold.

"We do everything we can to make it easy for the clients to get clean needles. Even go to people's homes if they are shy. But some clients cannot wait for us. For them the lack of syringes isn't the problem, the lack of drugs is the problem. It is easier if the clients have good relations with one another. That way, they can exchange for each other, and not everybody has to come to us every time."—*LALS*

LALS does HIV/AIDS counseling, drug counseling and referrals in the field and at the office and has recently added a family counseling component.

"Counseling is always one on one. Initially, when we tried it in a group, confidentiality was a problem and also everyone had different problems they wanted to discuss. It was impossible to focus on an individual, and without that you cannot make him satisfied. He needs to feel you are addressing his personal problem, not your problem, not the agency's agenda. Recently, we began counseling the IDU's family, too, and integrating them into the IDU's counseling. If the family can understand the IDU better—his addiction, what the HIV risks are—they can support him better and will also learn about HIV/AIDS.

"Drugs are very powerful and it is hard to make behavior change in this population. Some groups of IDUs, like street children, are harder to make aware of their health than others. Generally, IDUs are harder to motivate than other populations, and we think it takes about three years just to begin to get them to change their behavior consistently."—*LALS*

Half of LALS staff are medical workers, and they provide the IDUs and others with basic health care. Like other NGOs, LALS has found that their target population relies on them heavily for medications.

"I don't have time today. Maybe I will come to your office later, but can you give me some of that stuff for my sores right now?" —*Driver to CHOW in a taxi*

"This is one area where local people really like and support us, and this kind of contact brings us in touch with non-injecting drug users and others who need drug education and HIV information. The staff nurses carry medications and treat problems like burns, abscesses, coughs, syphilis, hepatitis. One of the most common problems is infections at the injection sites. For more serious problems, we take people to the hospital or clinic and after they come home our nurse provides medications and dressings until they are well. This is a costly program, but we feel it is important."—*LALS*

SOCIAL ACTION LEADS TO VULNERABILITY REDUCTION

Whether because of stigmatization, economic conditions, the effects of drug use or other factors, finding and keeping a job may be difficult for some IDUs. They may also neglect or be unable to pay for personal needs such as food, shelter and medical care, thus further increasing their vulnerability to HIV. Social awareness of their problems and needs is extremely low. There are only six drug treatment centers in Nepal, none of them residential, and they are overcrowded and offer few services. LALS' drug counseling program and its family counseling component help reduce vulnerability by providing support and by facilitating access to services. LALS' cordial relations with the police and narcotics bureaus, combined with its efforts to increase their awareness about drug addiction and HIV, also help protect some IDUs from repressive law enforcement. In addition, LALS has recently begun to develop a network for placing drug users in voluntary jobs at hospitals and with other organizations as a step towards integrating them into the community and raising community awareness.

EXPANDING PROGRAMS FOR IDUS

Organizations focusing on IDUs might consider the need for interventions outside the Kathmandu area and also look at ways to identify and reach possibly vulnerable sub-populations such as students, particular castes or ethnic groups and prisoners.

Programs that address IDUs' vulnerability to HIV strongly depend on cooperation from authorities to provide IDUs with services and protection from official harassment, and to prevent drug pushing. The kind of tension LALS has experienced with Nepal's authorities is on-going, and organizations targeting IDUs may want to build a response to this into their program design, addressing the need for continued awareness-raising around issues of legal and human rights.

Finally, education programs that can effectively bring these issues to the general population may help raise awareness and change public opinion in a constructive way.

SHAMBU PHITAL, CHOW

"I injected whatever I could get for 18 years. I went to prison for seven months and when I came out, I thought, this is my last chance. I had lost many things—my wife, my one child—they don't understand this. I was alone. I knew LALS when I was an addict, so I came and said, 'If I could get a job, I'll get out of drugs.' I'm out three and a half years now, but sometimes, when I see the addicts who were injecting with me... If I were not working here, I could go the wrong way. I have to be my own counselor now.

"My past helps me in my work. People I know from before respect me. They say, 'You were one of the worst junkies, now you are a gentleman, living with your family. How did you get like this?' I tell them, but then they say, 'For me, it is different. No family support, no job, I live on the street.' When I was an addict, I never wanted to hear what LALS was saying, that HIV was bigger than drugs and it would kill me before the drugs. Now, I give the same message and I believe it, but I know how hard it is to make them listen. Still, I think we are controlling it.

"Wherever I go, I hear from the community, 'These addicts are bad. Just let them die.' I explain how AIDS can come to anyone. It is hard to get the community to accept IDUs, even harder for the family. One person I know wanted to get off of drugs, but he didn't have any place to live. I convinced him to go with me to his family. His father says, 'I don't want this boy. I sent him to Korea for treatment, he came back and started again.' I took the father to another room and convinced him to give one more chance.

He saw I didn't look like a drug addict now, I looked like a social worker. So he took his son back. He is still there and he is changing day by day. Every week we go and give counseling. I don't know how long we will have to keep on. It is not that easy."

A MORNING WITH THE CHOWs

CHOW Shambu Phital, Staff Nurse Gita Ghatta and I leave
the LALS office one steamy morning and walk through a
miasma of pollution to a theater where LALS stops every
Tuesday and Thursday. Today there are four clients. A
young man agrees to talk to me, though he is clearly
uncomfortable. "If LALS weren't here we might not care.
You give us services, but if you didn't come, well...at least
we know about it [HIV]. But the new people wouldn't get
the message, and who knows who would tell them. I want
to have treatment and after that I want a job. If LALS could
provide that, a rehabilitation center for us after treatment...it would be better for us."

In our taxi to the next site we talk, in English, about needle exchange. The driver interrupts in Nepali to ask
Shambu about LALS and HIV. At our destination, the driver
asks for some medication, and Gita squeezes ointment into
a small plastic bag. Shambu urges him to come to LALS'
office. He saw the man's track marks when we got in the
taxi, Shambu tells me, but he would not have made the first
contact.

We cross a rubble- and garbage-strewn lot, and I wonder how Gita copes all day in her sari and delicate shoes.
Ten to 20 people meet here to inject, most are teenagers. A
man comes out of a tin and cardboard shack and exchanges
50 needles. He will sell those he does not use. Then two
women and four children emerge. A recent newborn has
disappeared, Gita says sadly. Both women are IDUs and sex
workers. The one who agrees to talk to me has a vicious

hangover, but rallies to stress that LALS has made a difference in her life. Like the other IDUs I've talked to, she has a vision of another life. "I've been interacting with LALS since 1991. I've learned a lot. Five of us girls took drug treatment once. I had TB, but now I'm OK. I want treatment again, and any kind of job so I don't *ever* have to come back here." Gita gives out medications and we move on to a quiet neighborhood where the clients come and go quickly. One is a well dressed man who had missed an earlier appointment with LALS. He catches up with us on the road and drops eight syringes into the yellow sharps container. Gita hands him eight more, two Band-Aids, a piece of cotton, a 35mm film container of bleach and some ointment. The CHOWs are less than half way through their day.

CHAPTER 9

UNCERTAIN HORIZONS:
LOOKING TOWARD THE FUTURE

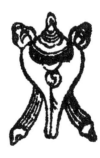

"AmFAR is trying to build Nepali organizations. With others it's OK; fund, staff the program, make the final report, finish. This is not going to happen with AmFAR, because many organizations will, I think, continue their programs. Maybe there will be some change in area or intensity, but it will continue."—*B. P. Memorial*

The HIV/AIDS epidemic in Nepal will continue to grow well into the foreseeable future, and skilled NGOs with close ties to their communities will be essential to the response. From the design phase of the project on, AmFAR has focused on developing the NGOs' ability to continue their work after AmFAR support ends.

One element of sustainability is to have strong organizations with the skills to monitor and evaluate both their community's needs and their own response to those needs, then direct and re-direct themselves on the basis of what they find. This is precisely what the AmFAR partner NGOs in this report describe themselves doing. This ability provides a firm foundation for facing the challenge of preventing the spread of HIV/AIDS in their communities. And it will be a challenge, particularly with respect to developing and implementing the interventions that are crucial to addressing the context of people's lives.

The NGO's present task, however, is to work to make their programs and their organizations sustainable so that they, and other organizations that will benefit from their experience, can meet these challenges. The AmFAR staff works with the grantees to develop their sustainability by enabling them to get grants from various donors, acquire visibility and develop networking. At bottom, however, sustainability requires that organizations be self-reliant in terms of making their own decisions, which is why AmFAR upholds the philosophy of empowering groups as opposed to merely providing them with funds for a set number of years. In the longer term, and it may never be possible in the context of Nepal, sustainability would also imply financial self-sufficiency. In a country where per capita income is just $160 a year, however, the NGOs will continue to need financial support from major donors well into the future.

SUSTAINING THE HIV/AIDS PROGRAMS

"Our aim is to sustain the program. To generate some income and to pass on our skills. We want to network in this region and apply the Nepalgung model, with the support of local organizations and groups. If we put our model elsewhere, we want to be able to transfer our knowledge and skills. That means developing our professionalism. And how can we sustain the institution without professional skills? As for income, condom social marketing might be a supportive activity. But this isn't the right time to try to be financially self-sufficient. Still, we are proud to be an organization with the *most* community contribution. For example, an NGO once took four Badi children to Kathmandu for school and the parents demanded compensation of 500 Rs a month from the NGO. The kids ran away and came home. Yet SAFE has a hostel where parents *pay us* 75 Rs a month to educate their kids. We established something needed in the community and the parents participate and pay. This is sustainability and community support."—*SAFE*

In mid 1995 the technical assistance staff organized a five day workshop on sustainability for the AmFAR NGOs. It emerged that the NGOs' primary concern is with sustaining their organizations while AmFAR hopes HIV/AIDS prevention programs will be sustained. According to Technical Advisor Paul Janssen, "These objectives are not mutually exclusive, but differing priorities have to be clarified to prevent misunderstanding." Community support is one key to sustaining both.

Bringing to the meeting all the lessons they had learned in the field, the participants stressed that the support of community leaders and detailed knowledge of community status, behaviors, attitudes, and values are critical for program success. Inadequate or inaccurate information could, they felt, spell failure. Many NGOs are making concrete efforts to involve the community in securing their programs' future. WOREC and NESCORD, for example, focus on building a strong base of volunteer AIDS educators from among community groups. SAFE hopes to motivate specific communities to support their own education. For example, they encourage the transport association to participate in and raise funds for SAFE's AIDS education booth at the bus park. Several NGOs train school and campus teachers to participate in providing AIDS education. And all the NGOs that have trained skilled peer educators have come to see them as WICOM does, as "the future main activists in the campaign for AIDS awareness."

NGOs are also working to become more cost effective and to develop sources of independent income for their programs. For example, ABC/Nepal, WOREC, NESCORD and others sell the IEC materials they produce and use the income to support their activities. Other NGOs charge for some of their services. BP Memorial charges a nominal fee at its STD clinic and NCWCA asks a small amount of NFE participants. "As such," says AmFAR Technical Advisor Paul Janssen, "these are good ideas. But if they lead to other (non-grantee) NGOs not being able to afford services, it undermines nationwide HIV prevention. Raising, discussing and solving issues like this are challenges for both NGOs and AmFAR and need a continuing dialogue."

As SAFE learned on the example of its hostel/school, programs that come up from the community (as opposed to being brought to the community) may get the most community participation and be most sustainable in the long run. Paul Janssen characterizes programs like this as "demand led," and says such services "are likely to create even more of a demand from the community, and there will always be a demand. If the NGO doesn't provide the service, people may create their own source or demand it from the government."

THE IMPORTANCE OF INTEGRATED HIV/AIDS PROGRAMS

"Before doing this work, I thought girl trafficking was caused by only one factor, and if the traffickers were put into prison, the problem would be solved. After four years of hard experience I see that it's not just a boy selling sweet dreams to girls. If a trafficker is imprisoned, and then tomorrow a political figure sets him free, the problem isn't solved. The political figures, the police force, the social workers should all be put together to work it out. But even that won't work unless we generate a very good income source for those people. Only one NGO working on this is not enough."—*MANK*

Given all the pressing issues in Nepal, community demand, at this stage, is not focused on HIV/AIDS services. After doing its initial needs assessment, one NGO reported back to AmFAR that people did not need condoms, they needed seeds. For an organization that focuses on AIDS prevention, not agricultural development, this kind of response can generate a certain tension. And given this tension, there may appear to be an inconsistency between what donors pose as a basic principle—to involve the community and respect its agenda—and the restrictions imposed by their mission or their policy makers. How, then, might the tension between condoms and seeds be resolved in a way that promotes the sustainability of HIV/AIDS programs?

One approach would be to work side by side with other INGOs and NGOs that have acquired expertise and have a commitment to social and economic development. Another approach would be to demonstrate even more clearly to target populations how activities such as NFE and income generation are necessary in order to lower vulnerability to HIV.

Programs that integrate HIV elements into a broader development context not only address a community's vulnerability to HIV, they are also most likely to be sustained with funding. Funding for development projects in general and for HIV programs in particular is drying up world wide, and donors want to achieve greater efficiency with fewer resources. "AIDS is becoming more critical in Nepal as resources are dwindling," says Keith Leslie of Save the Children/U.S. "If those resources are allocated for HIV prevention in consort with other development activities, the programs probably will survive longer. Only NGOs with a strong foundation will survive, and most of those are working in a broader based development perspective—with trafficking, economic development, a specific caste, etc. AIDS education will not stop trafficking, the economic problems are too severe. Bring it into a package of interventions where the whole family benefits, rather than one intervention which is hard for them to see as their most important public health hazard."

SUSTAINING THE ORGANIZATIONS

"At one time, NGOs here could be dollar farmers. They set up an organization and got a project. They had a signboard, but not performance. Now, such organizations find there is no way to survive. There is competition now among NGOs to become professional and have full time staff. They know how difficult it is to write proposals and convince donors."—*Anthropologist Ganesh Gurung*

"Since we developed this HIV program, we have all become better informed and much more educated, and we have developed a skill. Whoever we come in contact with, they get much more information and motivation from us than before. All the NGOs working in this field will have the same type of experience that we have had in manpower development."—*ICH*

AmFAR is working with the NGOs both to secure donor support and to reduce their dependency on it. In mid 1995, immediately after the five day sustainability workshop, AmFAR arranged a conference to bring the NGOs into direct contact with possible future support organizations. At the day-long event NGOs and INGOs discussed NGO support issues and shared their experiences, concerns and common expectations. Donors stressed the importance of paying close attention to identifying community needs, of looking at issues in a holistic way that would include multi-agency collaboration, and of professional management. The NGOs emphasized their need for more active involvement by support organizations in monitoring and providing technical assistance, and encouraged donors to understand the situation in Nepal and be flexible with respect to policy, program design and implementation. AmFAR's goal is to keep this kind of dialogue open and encourage the NGOs to develop strong programs for the future. "We are pushing the NGOs to look beyond NFE and income generation and think of other interventions, new activities," says Program Officer Azeliya Ranjitkar. "We provide skills training in proposal writing and have fund-raising workshops, but the organizations must also have a vision they can explain to the donor."

Continued dialogue may help both donors and NGOs avoid pitfalls such as the temptation on the part of NGOs to manipulate their objectives in order to meet donor guidelines. "One way to avoid this," says Paul Janssen, "is to build a donor/NGO dialogue first where the issues can be made explicit. Because if the goals do not really overlap, the project will not be sustainable. NGOs have to become more assertive toward support organizations, and I see that happening. BASE, for example, now refuses some grant offers and NNSWA is thinking hard about whether they are ready to scale up in order to work with a large donor. This is a sign of maturing."

THE EMERGING RESEARCH RESULTS: LESSONS FOR THE FUTURE

AmFAR's international program began with a simple research question: Can early intervention slow the spread of HIV in an low incidence country? It is far too early to evaluate the Nepal experience, but within a short period of time, a great deal of information has been collected from and by the NGOs using an organized or a logical approach to information gathering. This information was translated into program strategies or re-directions. There are a number of examples throughout this text of NGOs that made mistakes, approached people or the topic in an inappropriate way, went back and tried again until it worked better, and still keep refining their program. And *that* is the process of research: determining your mistakes and problems, suggesting solutions, testing those solutions. A lot of this has been going on throughout Nepal and a few primary lessons have emerged. These include:

- the recognition that no population is monolithic and therefore each population and each of its subsets requires a different approach—whether for sex education, for HIV information or for behavior change.

- the understanding that there is no substitute for knowing and having the trust of the community. There is little hard data about the health status, sexuality and sexual practices of Nepal's people, but the community can be the source of valuable information upon which to base interventions.

- the realization that there is a close synergy and interaction between risk-taking behaviors and contextual issues, and unless both are addressed together, HIV will find its way more forcefully into Nepal.

- the recognition, based on repeated experience, that programs that come from the community work, and therefore taking a grassroots approach is important.

- the understanding that monitoring and evaluation are crucial for determining community needs and measuring an organization's success in meeting them.

AmFAR, too, has learned valuable lessons, and Rev. Margaret Reinfeld, the former director of the international programs, thinks they have value for funders and researchers alike. "We learned important things about how to do funding. With only a small number of decision makers in charge, implementation was very quick and we had a level of oversight rarely enjoyed in international work. And that oversight gave us flexibility in terms of budget and program modification. Also, we were willing to live with ragged edges. It's not going to work if you don't give people the space to learn from their mistakes and experience. In addition, the long-term, non-competitive nature of the funding really helped build up a grantee network, and some of the traditional divisions of Nepal society began to fade. Brahmin ladies work with untouchables. They feel a common purpose and that is important for a society. It's an important part of what we did.

"We could not have done this without having AIDS expertise. The programs may look straightforward, but they are complicated undertakings. You have to wed the research, the AIDS expertise and the organizational development. The important research lesson is that you have to have a multiple methodology approach and be very clear that a lot of the answers coming from the program won't be quantitative. You can't count beans. You have to take a longitudinal look at organizations, see whole communities as a unit of analysis. And you develop your research along with the people involved, teach them research methodologies. Otherwise, you haven't done your job, because you haven't left anything behind they can use."

WILL THE AmFAR NGOs IMPACT THE COURSE OF HIV/AIDS IN NEPAL?

It has been the experience with the HIV/AIDS pandemic that change, whether behavioral or attitudinal, is difficult and occurs only in small steps. To date, the AmFAR program has taken several steps—some of them quite significant—to bring about awareness and change. On the institutional level, it has facilitated potentially valuable coordination among organizations responsible for addressing HIV/AIDS in Nepal. It has also empowered community-based individuals and groups to take ownership of the response to the pandemic—as SAFE puts it, "to motivate for self-help." LALS has documented no new HIV cases among its client IDU population in two years. The Badi scx workers have dramatically increased their condom use and reduced their STD and pregnancy rates. MANK and WOREC report a sharp decrease in trafficking where their programs are active, though it has increased in surrounding villages. Peer educators in some schools have the unprecedented ability to provide their fellow students with factual information about HIV/AIDS and STDs.

In addition, the response to HIV by the AmFAR partner NGOs, and other NGOs and INGOs, has brought some changes in the focus of development work and NGO work in Nepal. It has increased the focus on human rights issues such as confidentiality, privacy and individual rights, on some underprivileged groups, and on trafficking to India and prostitution in Nepal. In a context where people's needs are overwhelming in every field, continued monitoring of where HIV develops may help identify people and groups that are particularly vulnerable not only to the virus, but to other health issues and social problems as well. It is often difficult to define where stigmatization or discrimination exists against certain communities or sub-populations within them. It may be easier in the long run to identify where HIV has found its niches, and where there is HIV, there must be, or have been, discrimination.

This may be as true elsewhere as in Nepal. AmFAR's Mary McMechan, who has worked closely with the Nepal projects from the outset, thinks that the lessons learned in Nepal may be broadly useful. "Working in the cultural context of different populations that are disadvantaged, discriminated against, I've found that, despite the presumed differences among them in HIV prevention, there are common themes throughout. The 15-year-old girl trafficked to a brothel or the one exposed to gangs on the street in the Bronx—I don't see a difference. The 'cultures' are different—but whose culture is it? The girls'? The risk factors, how high they are, why people are exposed to them—it seems to me those issues are identical. All the lessons drawn from Nepal may be relevant to AmFAR's mission in the U.S. And the experience of the NGOs we work with in the States—experience gained by testing their assumptions and going back to the community and being accountable to it—has been affirmed in a new setting. Despite their different professional capacities, the NGOs in the U.S. and in Nepal are equally able to know their community and the source of whatever puts it at greatest risk."

Another commonality is that NGOs in both the U.S. and Nepal are facing sharply reduced funding. Mary McMechan characterizes it as donor fatigue based on "having to switch from thinking 'we're going to beat this soon' to looking at planning for the next 50 years." For Nepal's NGOs, the shortfall cannot be made up by angels, benefits or profit-making projects, and the country's scarcity of skills, resources and funds makes this is a critical period. There is no way Nepal can respond to its emerging epidemic of HIV/AIDS and stabilize the gains already made without continued international support. It is one thing for a

Nepali girl to tell a visiting American that she will slap anyone who tries to traffick her. It is quite another thing to initiate, support and sustain the social and economic changes needed to make sure she is not forced into sex work despite her courage.

NGO NETWORKS AND COORDINATION

"We have crossed to a new stage now where we have to sit down together and decide how we can build a strong AIDS education program. Every year, we will need a better impact and more and more programs. If we stay in the stage where we are, we will not have this impact. I don't have a formula for how to do it and how to be sustainable. But it may happen when we all get together—NGOs, donors, the government—to talk nationwide about what we need."—*ICH*

When AmFAR designed its international program, developing organizational networks and involving government leaders were considered important components for success and sustainability. Neither plan evolved exactly as planned. NGO networking is valuable because organizations can share information and scarce resources and avoid duplication of services. Cooperative NGO/government links foster determining and implementing the most effective distribution of responsibility for meeting the challenge of HIV/AIDS.

But AmFAR technical assistance staff found that coordination among NGOs cannot be imposed. Informal coordination in which NGOs provide one another with resource people or participate in each others trainings have worked best. Formal networking has been less successful. AmFAR has tried to establish non-hierarchical NGO networks based on similar focuses and target populations, and several meetings have been held. "AmFAR's role,"

Paul Janssen has concluded, "should be to capitalize on networking opportunities as they arise."

AmFAR itself coordinated very successfully with the government's National AIDS Program in year one, but interaction has fallen off, due, in large part, to NAP's long-term lack of a permanent director. Former NAP Director Dr. B.B. Karki had hoped to foster more cooperation, but it wasn't possible in his short tenure. Dr. Karki feels that the National Program should play a leadership role to coordinate the HIV/AIDS programs rather than take up activities itself, but he laments the lack of coordination among the various players. "The role of the INGOs should be not just to support the NGOs but to coordinate with the National Program. And if INGOs could do that, then naturally the NGOs they support would too. The organizations coordinated by AmFAR were closer to me and used to interact freely, but others had the attitude 'Why should I bother about you? Your program does not support me with money.' They should bother because it benefits all. If the epidemic breaks out in some area, the National Program will go in, and if an NGO is working in that area, everyone will need to cooperate."

PARTNER NGOS STRIVE TOWARD SUSTAINABILITY AFTER EARLY END OF AMFAR FUNDING

At the close of 1995, AmFAR and its partner NGOs had to face the realization that, following a growing global trend, AmFAR could not raise the funds to support the final six months of the three year project. In response, AmFAR and the technical assistance team accelerated a series of programs and workshops for the NGOs designed to focus on issues of sustainability and strategic planning for the future. (The first of these programs, presented in mid-1995, is described in Chapter 9.) The workshops not only focused on skills such as assessing organizational strengths and weaknesses and developing strong proposals, they also provided an ideal opportunity for representatives of donor agencies and NGOs to meet and interact. In the light of the NGOs' need to find substitute funding quickly, this exposure proved invaluable.

Clearly, the prospect of doing HIV/AIDS work with experienced, trained Nepali organizations was very attractive to donors. Of the 16 NGOs, all but one (NESCORD) have found sufficient funding to continue their organizations, and all but one of those (CRDS) will continue doing HIV/AIDS work in either vertical or integrated programs. These NGOs can be divided into two general "types" of organizations: "community based," on the one hand and "service delivery" on the other. The former tend to come up from a community, involve it in decision making and design programs in response to their needs. The latter tend to be more professional, make top down decisions and do not have a clear constituency. They bring a skilled service to communities they believe have a need for it. As almost all the NGOs have been funded for 1996, donors are clearly interested in both NGO approaches. And as nearly all NGOs will continue with HIV/AIDS programs, it is clear that not only donors, but also the communities are convinced that addressing Nepal's emerging epidemic is a true community need.

AmFAR's initial objective was to initiate a community-based response to HIV/AIDS in Nepal and study the effect of that response in a low incidence country. Almost three years later, as 14 of the original 17 NGOs continue to provide communities with increasingly well crafted HIV/AIDS programs, it is fair to say that that initial objective was achieved—thanks in large measure to the extraordinary perseverance and dedication of the NGOs.

HIV/AIDS, HEALTH AND HUMAN RIGHTS

The linkage of AIDS, health, and human rights is profoundly important. AIDS has brought us to the threshold of
a new understanding of health and society. Through the
struggle with AIDS in communities in Nepal and other
countries around the world, we have seen that vulnerability
to HIV is above all societally determined. We now know that
regardless of where and in which community HIV first
enters a population, it will find its way inexorably to those
who were already discriminated against, marginalized, and
stigmatized before the appearance of AIDS.

Public health programs that do not understand or deal
directly with the societal dimensions of vulnerability are
condemned to remain of limited effectiveness. Public
health measures, as traditionally defined and as reflected in
ongoing AIDS programs, cannot make up for the factors
borne out of the societal environment that lead to
increased vulnerability.

There is more to the societal context of health than
income, employment status and educational level. A more
comprehensive and coherent vision of societal vulnerability
is attained by linking our understanding of public health
with human rights. For to realize human rights, as articu-
lated in the Universal Declaration of Human Rights, is to
ensure the underlying conditions which people need to be
healthy.

Two paths lie before us. One is the path that holds fast
to traditional public health ideas and approaches which are
necessary and important, but manifestly not sufficient to

deal with HIV/AIDS. The other is a more difficult, complex, and challenging path that requires us to address the root causes—the societal causes—of ill health and premature death.

To connect human rights with public health, we need to work with those already striving to promote and protect human rights and dignity within each society. This work is as concrete as any work in public health. Starting with an analysis of the status of respect for human rights and dignity in our own societies, we can discover how the failure to realize certain specific rights can lead to increased vulnerability to HIV/AIDS. Then we can work to reduce that vulnerability by combining AIDS-specific programs with activism and targeted efforts to realize those rights.

The societal vulnerability which underlies HIV/AIDS is common to many, if not most, of the major health problems. Our collective, pioneering work linking promotion and protection of health with promotion and protection of human rights thus opens new avenues in understanding and advancing human well-being in the world.

Jonathan Mann, MD, MPH
François-Xavier Bagnoud Professor
of Health and Human Rights,
and Professor of Epidemiology
and International Health
Harvard School of Public Health

BIBLIOGRAPHY

This bibliography (1990-1995) is intended as a resource for all those engaged in designing community-based health and social programs in Nepal. It is hoped that, by building on existing knowledge, future programs will be enhanced and sustained for the better lives of Nepali communities.

1990:

Child Workers in Nepal—Concerned Group (CWIN), *Lost Childhood: A Survey Research on Street Children of Kathmandu* (18 pp): CWIN, Kathmandu, Nepal, 1990.

B. M. Devkota et al., *Siraha District Baseline Study in Muksar, Lalpur, Jamdaha, Phulkahakatti, Honumannagar and Ayodhyanagar* (87 pp): Save the Children (STC) (US), Kathmandu, Nepal, 1990.

G. Ferster, *A framework of analysis for outreach delivery of FP and MCH services from health post to households in Nepal* (technical report): The World Bank, Washington, DC, December 1990.

D. Ghimire, *Chelibeti Ko Abaidh Byapara Yesaka Bibidh Paksha* (Nepali): ABC/Nepal, Kathmandu, Nepal, 1990.

Integrated Development System (IDS), *Improving Family Planning Acceptance Through Panchayat Based Clinics and Community Women Volunteers* (59 pp): The FPAN/CEDPA, Kathmandu, Nepal, 1990.

J. T. Maag et al., *Evaluation of Natural Family Planning Programme in IHDP (Dolakha) and FPAN (Kathmandu Valley)*: SDC/N Ministry of Health (MOH), Kathmandu, Nepal, 1990.

T. M. Malaby, "The pluralism of illness beliefs in Nepal: a theoretical appraisal," B. A. Thesis, Harvard University, Cambridge, MA, 1990.

Nepal Population and Health Project, Outreach service delivery, health post and below (draft), Kathmandu, Nepal: Nepal Population and Health Project, Working Group I, April 1990.

New Era, *Acceptors' Verification Study of Nepal Red Cross Family Planning and Primary Health Care Project* (63 pp): Family Planning International Assistance (FPIA), Bangkok, Thailand, 1990.

New Era, *Baseline Study on Health Status in Sindhuli District*: IHDP and SDC/Nepal, Kathmandu, Nepal, 1990.

New Era, *A Comparative Impact Evaluation of the UNICEF Assisted Semi-Urban Sanitation Pilot Programme and the East Consultant's Sanitation Action Programme*: United Nations Children's Fund (UNICEF)/Nepal, Kathmandu, Nepal, 1990.

New Era, *Health Survey in Dolakha District* (138 pp): IHDP/SDC Jawalakhel, Lalitpur, Nepal, 1990.

New Era, *Impact Study of Family Planning and Child Health Project*: Japan International Cooperation Agency (JICA), Kathmandu, Nepal, 1990.

New Era, *A Study on Family Planning Adoption and Health Care in Majhigaon and Dummrechaur Villages of Sindhupalchowk District Nepal*: World Neighbors, Kathamndu, Nepal, 1990.

New Era, *Verification of Natural Family Planning Acceptors' Data*: SDC, Lalitpur, Nepal, 1990.

M. S. Rajbhandari and J. T. Maag, *The User's Point of View on Natural Family Planning Programme in the Dolakha District*

(IHDP//SDC) and Kathmandu Valley (FPAN): MAAG, Kathmandu, Nepal, 1990.

A. Shrestha, T. T. Kane, and H. Hamal, "Contraceptive social marketing in Nepal: consumer and retailer knowledge, needs and experience," *Journal of Biosocial Science* 22(1990):305-322.

L. P. Upreti, *Benighat Health Post Case Study* (37 pp): The John Snow Public Health Group (JSI), Kathmandu, Nepal, 1990.

Valley Research Group (VaRG), *A Follow-up Study on Depoprovera Acceptors* (Draft Report) (77 pp): United Nations Fund for Population Activities (UNFPA), Pulchowk, Lalitpur, Nepal, 1990.

1991:

R. K. Adhikari, *Trends in Nutritional Status in Nepal Since 1975* (74 pp): UNICEF, Kathmandu, Nepal, 1991.

C. Arnold, "Nepal: project entry point" in: *Child care: meeting the needs of working mothers and their children*, A. Leonard and C. Landers, eds. (New York, NY: Seeds, 1991): 5-13.

Y. P. Bhagat, "A Comparative Study on Rural and Urban Mothers Regarding Knowledge Attitude and Practice of Formula Feeding in Bara District": Nepal Institute of Medicine (IOM)/Central Campus, Maharajgunj, Nepal, 1991.

B. K. Bhatta et al., *Community Field Report of Tatopani* (for IOM pre-medicine course) (19 pp): IOM, Kathmandu, Nepal, 1991.

S. B. Chaudhary, *Review and analysis of NEP/88/P17, Strengthening health manpower training for the delivery of primary health care services through Regional Training Centers*: prepared for the UNFPA, New York, NY, August 1991.

Centre for Women and Development (CWD), *Prostitution in Relation to Socio-economic and Health Problems (A Case Study of Badi Community)* (50 pp): World Health Organization (WHO)/MOH, Kathmandu, Nepal, 1991.

Child Worker in Nepal—Concerned Group (CWIN), *Child Labour in the Tea Estates of Nepal*: CWIN, Kathmandu, Nepal, 1991.

COWI Consult, Effectiveness of multilateral agencies at country level (case studies), Copenhagen, Denmark: Danish International Development Agency (DANIDA), 1991.

D. Hinrichsen, "Nepal—struggling for a common future," *Populi* 18 (1991): 43-51.

Integrated Development System (IDS), *Knowledge, Attitude and Practice Towards Health and Essential Drugs in Rural Nepal* (106 pp): UNICEF, Kathmandu, Nepal, 1991.

Interface PVT Ltd., *A Baseline Survey of Population/Family Welfare Programme for Woman Through PCRW of WDS/MLD* (182 pp): UNICEF/Nepal, Kathmandu, Nepal, 1991.

M. G. Killer, *Tibetan Women and Children in Nepal A Preliminary Report on the Conditions Effecting the Health and Welfare Status of the Tibetan Community in Nepal*: UNICEF, Kathmandu, Nepal, 1991.

I. Khanal, *A Study on Causative failure of Burn and Syndrome Among the Staff Nurse in TUTH* (for Partial Fulfillment of BSc Nursing, Institute of Medicine) (29 pp): T.U., Nursing Campus, Maharajgunj, Nepal, 1991.

D. Malla and A. Shrestha, *Based on 100 percent Population Registration and Baseline Survey of Maternal and Child Health Ilaka No. 1 Gorkha District* (59 pp): STC (US), Kathmandu, Nepal, 1991.

B. Maskey , M. Levitt and M. Simpson-Hebert, *Maternal and Child Health: Management Issues at Community Health Post and District Level*:: Division of Nursing, Ministry of Health (MOH), commissioned by SCF/UK, Kathmandu, Nepal 1991.

Ministry of Labour and Social Welfare (MOLSW), Women Development Division, *Report of National Tripartite Workshop on the role of labour administration in promotion of employment and welfare of women in Nepal*: Kathmandu, Nepal: ILO/ARPLA /MOLSW, 1991.

New Era, *A Baseline Study on Health Status in Ramechhap District* (121 pp): IHDP/SDC, Jawalakhel, Lalitpur, Nepal, 1991.

New Era, *A Report on the Traditional Birth Attendants Training Programme*: Jiri Technical Schools/SDC, Lalitpur, Nepal, 1991.

M. R. Pandey, N. M. Daulaire, E. S. Starbuck et al., "Reduction in total under-five mortality in western Nepal through community-based antimicrobial treatment of pneumonia," *Lancet* 338(1991): 993-997.

R. Pradhan et al., *Community Field Report of Banskhark VDC of Sindhupalchok District for Pre-medicine Course to IOM* (32 pp): T.U., IOM, TUTH, Kathmandu, Nepal, 1991.

P. R. Rajbhandari, *Review and analysis of NEP/88/P03, Strengthening health network with community participation for MCH/FP*, New York, NY: prepared for UNFPA, July 1991.

Research and Study Centre (P) Ltd., Kamaladi, *An Assessment of the Rural Family Welfare Project at Rupandehi, Kanchanpur and Surkhet Branches* (71 pp): Nepal Family Planning Association, Kathmandu, Nepal, 1991.

Save the Children Fund (UK), *Annual Report 1990-1991*.

H. Singh, *Restructuring of health services in Nepal* (interim report), Geneva, Switzerland: World Health Organization, 1991.

Valley Research Group (VaRG), *Operation Research on Women's Involvement in MCH/FP Services* (127 pp): UNFPA, Pulchowk, Lalitpur, Nepal, 1991.

Valley Research Group (VaRG), *A follow-up Study on Depoprovera Acceptors* (82 pp), UNFPA, Pulchowk Lalitpur, Nepal, 1991.

E. E. Whitney and M. W. Lediard, *Nepal: developing decentralized IEC programs*, Kathmandu, Nepal, December 16-28: USAID, Johns Hopkins, unpublished, 1991.

WOREC, *A Report of the Seminar on Socio-economic Aspect of HIV/AIDS in Nepal* (51 pp): United Nations Development Program (UNDP)/Nepal, Kathmandu, Nepal, 1991.

C. Write, *Five Years of Community Mental Health Services—An Evaluation Report*: WMN, Kathmandu, Nepal, 1991.

1992:

W. G. Axinn, "Rural income-generating programs amd fertility limitation: evidence from a microdemographic study in Nepal," *Rural Sociology* 57(1992): 396-413.

S. Basnet et al., *Study Report on Effectiveness of Mother-craft Teaching to Selected Primigravida Mothers at T.U. Teaching Hospital* (TUTH): TUTH, Kathmandu, Nepal, 1992.

H. Bongartz, F. E. Stiftung, and The Nepal Foundation for Advanced Studies (seminar papers), *Foreign aid and the role of NGOs in the development process of Nepal*, The Nepal Foundation for Advanced Studies in cooperation with F. E. Stiftung: Kathmandu, Nepal, 1992.

Centre for Women and Development (CWD), *Child Nutrition Survey* (124 pp): K-BIRD, Kathmandu, Nepal, 1992.

M. Dupal and C. Carter, *Report on Baseline Survey of Siraha District, Child Survival VII Project* (65 pp): Save the Children (STC) (US), Kathmandu, Nepal, 1992.

M. Dupar, *Report of Jeevan Jal Preparation Survey* (30 pp): STC (US), Kathmandu, Nepal, 1992.

M. Dupar, *Report of Community Health Volunteer and Mothers' Groups Literacy Survey* (14 pp): STC (US), Kathmandu, Nepal, 1992.

A. Frederick et al., *Rural Social Marketing Project in Gorkha; Sales Survey Report* (131 pp): STC (US), Kathmandu, Nepal, 1992.

B. R. Gyawali, *Demographic and Socio-economic Impact on Fertility of Sarki Community, A Case Study of Thanpati Village in Gulmi District* (Dissertation) (82 pp): T.U., Kirtipur, Nepal, 1992.

W. Hoff, "Traditional healers and community health," *World Health Forum* 13 (1992): 182-187.

Institute of Integrated Development System (IIDS), *Schooling and Maternal Behaviour in Rural Nepal: Pathways to Child Survival and Health* (18 pp): The Ford Foundation, New Delhi, India, 1992.

L. P. Kak and S. Narasimhan, *The impact of family planning employment on field workers' lives: a strategy for measuring empowerment* (technical report), Washington, DC: Center for Development and Population Activities (CEDPA),1992.

S. Khanal, *Desired Family Size: A Case Study of Rupse VDC* (A dissertation): T.U. Kirtipur, Nepal, 1992.

K. Laslie et al., *AIDS Education and Prevention Project Among Tamang and Lower Caste Communities in Nuwakot District of Central Nepal* (Proposal): STC (US), 1992.

S. Mabin, Save the Children Fund, Nepal, *Chautara Project Health Facility Programme:* An Overview, Save the Children Fund (UK): Lalitpur, Nepal, 1992.

S. Neupane, *A Study on Breast Feeding Status in Rural and Urban Areas of Central Development Region, Nepal* (37 pp): UNICEF, Kathmandu, Nepal, 1992.

National Planning Commission (NPC), *Eastern Regional Planning Office Dhankuta, Service Centre Location Analysis and Rural*

Development of Case Study of Illam District: NPC, Regional Office, Dhankuta, Nepal, 1992.

S. Onta, *Environmental Degradation and its Impact on Health of Bhutanese Refugees in Jhapa* (74 pp): Resource Center for Primary Health Care, Bagbazar, Kathmandu, Nepal, 1992.

B. Rai et al., *District Public Health and Demographic Profile of Sindhupalchok District (submitted to IOM for partial fulfillment of BPH)* (57 pp): T.U., Department of Community Medicine, Central Campus, Maharajgunj, Nepal, 1992.

C. Sharma et al., *Report of Focus Group Discussion: Immunization Control of Diarrhoeal Diseases of Acute Respiratory Infection (Siraha District)* (44 pp): STC (US), Kathmandu, Nepal, 1992.

G. Subedi, *Determinants of Contraceptive Use of Case Study at Chaturale Village, Nuwakot* (dissertation for partial fulfillment of MA) (98 pp): T.U., Kirtipur, Nepal, 1992.

Valley Research Group (VaRG), *An Evaluation of FP/MCH Services Delivery Support Project* (145 pp): UNFPA, Pulchowk, Lalitpur, Nepal, 1992.

1993:

P. Bhatt P, V. L. Gurubacharya and G. Vadies, "A unique community of family-oriented prostitutes in Nepal uninfected by HIV-1," *International Journal of STD and AIDS* 4(1993):280-283.

C. N. Chaulagai, "Urban community health workers," *World Health Forum* 14 (1993): 16-19.

Family Planning Association of Nepal (FPAN) University Research Corperation, "Improving family planning acceptance through panchayat based clinics and outreach services" in: *Operations research family planning database project summaries*, New York, NY: compiled by The Population Council, 1993.

K. R. Gautam, *Pre-implementation (Base Line) Survey on AIDS Education and Support Programme at Damak and Dharan municipalities and Itahari VDC* (30 pp): Nepal Society for Community and Rural Development Center (NESCORD), Kathmandu, Nepal, 1993.

Institute of Community Health (ICH), *Project Report on AIDS Education and Prevention Program, Tikapur, Kailali* (60 pp): STC (US), Kathmandu, Nepal, 1993.

Institute of Community Health (ICH), *Project Report on AIDS and Prevention Program (Tikapur, Kailali, Western Region)*: STC (US), Kathmandu, Nepal, 1993.

A. R. Joshi, "Maternal schooling and child health: new evidence from a community-level study in rural Nepal," Qualifying paper for Harvard Graduate School of Education, Harvard University, Cambridge, MA, 1993.

T. Kuratsuji, "The joint JMA-JICA project in Nepal," *Acta Pædiatrica Japonica* 35 (1993): 571-575.

MOH/Central Region Health Directorate (CRHD) Pulchowk, *Lalitpur, Assessment of Female Community Health Volunteer Programme in Bara, Makawanpur, Nuwakot and Rammechhap District (Report)*: MOH/CHRD, Pulchowk, Lalitpur, Nepal, 1993.

New Era, *Diagnostic Assess of the Female Community Health Volunteer Programme in Nepal*: The Population Council Asia and Near East Operations Research and Technical Assistance Project, Kathmandu, Nepal, 1993.

New Era et al., *Nepal Fertility, Family Planning and Health Survey* (180 pp): MOH, Kathmandu, Nepal 1993.

R. Rajbhandary, *Present Status of Nepalese Prostitutes in Bombay (Survey Report)* (13 pp): Women's Rehabitation Centre (WOREC) Kathmandu, Nepal, 1993.

J. G. Rimon 2d and M. Lediard, *Nepal: IEC needs assessment—findings and recommendations* (technical report), Baltimore, MD: Johns Hopkins School of Public Health, Center for Communication Programs, Population Communication Services, 1993.

J. Rowley, "Bhorletar: the sustainable village," *People and the Planet* 2(1993): 14-19.

I. Singh et al., *Study on the effects of Socio-economic Condition and Cultural Beliefs and Attitudes of Mothers on their Awareness About Child Spacing and Fertility*: IOM, Family Health Centre, T.U., Kathmandu, Nepal, 1993.

H. Shrestha et al., *Report of the Study of the Impact of Counselling Service on the Acceptance and Continuation of Temporary Contraceptive Measures*: Human Reproduction Project Department of Community Medicine, IOM, Maharajgunj, Nepal, 1993.

I. Smith, "Tuberculosis control learning games," *Tropical Doctor* 23(1993):101-103.

J. Thapa, *Study on Marketing of Depoprovera in Nepal Through Private Sector* (71 pp): UNFPA, Lalitpur, Nepal, 1993.

R. Thapaliya, *Child Survival and Baseline Survey Reports, Ilaka 1, 12 and 13 Far-eastern Nuwakot District* (126 pp): STC (US) Kathmandu, Nepal, 1993.

G. Toffin, *The anthropology of Nepal, from tradition to modernity*, proceedings of the Franco-Nepalese Seminar held in the French Cultural Center, Kathmandu, Nepal 18-20 March 1992: French Cultural Center, French Embassy, 1993.

1994:

Anonymous, "Community health workers—experiences in three countries," *Alternatives* 1(1994): 10-11.

Anonymous, "Continuing product development," *CRS News* 9(1994): 1-4.

Anonymous, "People readily pay for quality services in Nepal," *JOICFP News* 246 (1994): 6.

Anonymous, "SOMARC and CRS social marketing expansion to long-term method (injectable)," *CRS News* 9 (1994): 3.

Backward Society Education (BASE), *Tharu Education for Transformation, Third Year Report*: DANIDA 1994.

M. Bhatterai, "Using local resources to fight HIV/AIDS in Nepal," *AIDS Captions* 1(1994)13-15.

D. Caudill, "Beyond Cairo: the integration of population and environment in Baudha-Bahunipati, Nepal" (pamphlet), Oklahoma City, OK: World Neighbors, 1994.

Central Regional Health Service Directorate, Ministry of Health (MOH), HMG, *Assessment of Female Community Health Volunteer Programme in Sindhupalchok and Parsa Districts*: HMG, MOH, Kathmandu, Nepal, 1994.

T. Cox and B. K. Subedi, *Sexual Networking in Five Urban Areas in the Nepal Terai, An Assessment of AIDS and STDs*: Prevention Network Valley Research Group, Kathmandu, Nepal, 1994.

T. Cox and B. K. Subedi, *Sexual Networking in Five Urban Areas of Southern Nepal* (62 pp): AIDSCAP, Kathmandu, Nepal, 1994.

Clark University USA and Institute of Integrated Development System (IIDS), *Managing Resources in a Nepalese Village: Changing Dynamics of Gender Caste and Ethnicity* (50 pp): Clark University, Worcester, Massachusetts, USA, 1994.

Centre for Women and Development (CWD), *Preliminary Study on Children-At-Risk in Narayanghat, Children-at-Risk*: NWG, Dillibazar, Kathmandu, Nepal, 1994.

M. Dupar, *Child Survival VII, Final Knowledge, Practice and Coverage Survey (Siraha District)* (30 pp): STC (US), Kathmandu, Nepal, 1994.

S. Fuller et al., *A Study of Children and Disease in Gorkha District* (24 pp): STC (US), Kathmandu, Nepal, 1994.

Institute of Integrated Development System (IIDS), *Baseline KAP Survey on Sustainable Community Based FP/MCH Project with Special Focus on Women in Sunsari District* (III pp): Japanese Organization for International Co-operation in Family Planning Inc by IIDS, Kathmandu, Nepal, 1994.

Institute of Integrated Development System (IIDS), *Determinants of Abortion* and *Subsequent Reproductive Behaviour Among Women of Three Urban Districts of Nepal* (152 pp and 246 pp): Development and Research Training in Human Reproduction, WHO, Kathmandu, Nepal, 1994.

U. Karmacharya, *Impact Study of Ilaka 1 Programme Gorkha District First Study Visit Report* (31 pp): STC (US), Kathmandu, Nepal, 1994.

S. Maharjan et al., *A Study on the KABP and HIV Prevalence Among Injecting Drug Users in Nepal WAVC 4* (36 pp): Life Saving & Life Giving Society (LALS), Kathmandu, Nepal, 1994.

D. Malla, *Report of Village Health Register up-dating Survey* (6 pp): STC (US), Kathmandu, Nepal, 1994.

Nepal Netra Jyoti Sangh, *A Study on Present Status and Future Prospects* (186 pp): Kathmandu, Nepal 1994.

New Era, *A follow-up Survey of IUD Acceptors'* HMG/MOH/Family Health Division: SDC, Lalitpur, Nepal, 1994.

New Era, *Status of Contraceptive Supplies in Selected Districts of Nepal*: HMG/MOH/Family Health Division, Kathmandu, Nepal, 1994.

New Era, *Xerophthalmia Prevalence Survey in Five Districts of Far and Mid-Western Region of Nepal, Vitamin A Field Support Project (VITAL)*: International Science & Technology Institute Inc

1616 North Fort Myer Drive, Suit 1240, Arlington, VA 22209, USA, 1994.

S. Onta, *Gender Differences of Morbidity and Case Study of Khanchowk Health Post, Enhancement of Research Capacity in Nepal*: A Primary Health Care Project, Kathmandu, Nepal, 1994.

B. Paudel, *The Study on Knowledge and Attitude About HIV/AIDS Amongst School Teachers of A Rural Area Nepal Rupandehi, Community Medicine Dept*: IOM Central Campus, Maharajgunj, Nepal, 1994.

K. Paudel, *A Study on the Causes of Low Oral Pills Contraception Among the Acceptors in Thecho VDC, Lalitpur (A Research Paper as a Partial Fulfillment of the Requirements of Bachelors Degree in Public Health)*: IOM, Department of Medicine, T.U., Maharajgunj, Nepal, 1994.

A. F. Purdey, G. B. Adhikari, S. A. Robinson et al., "Participatory health development in rural Nepal: clarifying the process of community empowerment," *Health Education Quarterly* 21 (1994) 329-343.

S. C. Regmi and R. K. Adhikari, *A Study on the Factors Influencing Nutritional Status of Adolescent Girls* (139 pp): New ERA, Kathmandu, Nepal, 1994.

Research Centre for Integrated Development, Nepal (RECID/N), *An Evaluation on the Impact of AIDS Education and Awareness Programme*: Child Development Society, American Foundation for AIDS Research (AmFAR) Project, Kathmandu, Nepal, 1994.

J. Robertson et al., *Report on Nutrition Survey Siraha District* (25 pp): STC (US), Kathmandu, Nepal, 1994.

S. Subba and S. Subha, *CWIN report—Chantiers Jeunes Observation Study on the Status of Girl Children in Nepal with Special Reference to Khokana VDC and Bungmati VDC Ward No. 9*: BALIKA/CWIN, Kathmandu, Nepal, 1994.

M. Thapa, *Action Research on Women's Participation and Leadership in Mental Health and Family Planning*: IOM/MOH/WHO/United Nation Fund for Population Activities (UNFPA), Kathmandu, Nepal, 1994.

S. Tipping, *Summary of Nepal DMPA marketing research findings*, unpublished, 1994.

Valley Research Group (VaRG), *Condom, Oral, and Injectable Users Profile Study in Nepal* (136 pp): SOMARC/The Futures Group, Washington, DC, USA, 1994.

Valley Research Group (VaRG), *CRS Consumer KAP Tracking Study Among Men and Women in Nepal* (145 pp): SOMARC/The Futures Group, Washington, DC, USA, 1994.

J. Wakil, *A Study on AIDS Knowledge and AIDS Related Practices Among Migrant Labourer of Matsari VDC Rautahat* (41 pp): T.U. Institute of Medicine, Community Medicine Department, Maharajgunj, Nepal, 1994.

Women's Rehabilitation Centre (WOREC), *Annual report* 1992-1993, Kathmandu, Nepal: WOREC, 1994.

The World Bank, Population and Family Health Project—March 1994 (staff appraisal report #10812-NEP), Washington, DC: The World Bank, 1994.

1995:

Anonymous, "Quality care for community-based FP/MCH," *JOICFP News* 248 (1995): 1.

Centre for Women and Development (CWD), *Video Film on Girl Trafficking and AIDS*: CCO, Kathmandu, Nepal, (released) 1995.

C. N. Chaulagai, "Community financing for essential drugs in Nepal," *World Health Forum* 16 (1995): 92-94.

F. Curtale, B. Siwakoti, C. Lagrosa et al., "Improving Skills and Utilization of Community Health Volunteers in Nepal," *Social Science & Medicine* 40(1995): 1117-1125.

B. R. Devkota, *A Mid-term Review Report on AIDS Awareness and Education Programmefor Industrial Workers and People of Sainik Basti, Kaski*: Manavothan, Kathmandu, Nepal, 1995.

I. Onozaki and T. M. Shakya, "Feasibility study of a district tuberculosis control program with an 8-month short-course chemotherapy regimen utilizing the integrated health service network under field conditions in Nepal," *Tubercle & Lung Disease* 76(1995): 65-71.

New Era, *A Baseline Study of Commercial Sex Workers and Sex Clients on the Land Transportation Routs from Naubise to Janakpur and Birgunj*: AIDSCAP Family Health International, Ramshah Path, Kathmandu, Nepal, 1995.

New Era, *Evaluation of SCF Traditional Healers (Dhami-Jhankri) Training Programme*: Save the Children Fund (UK), Patan Dhoka, Lalitpur, Nepal, 1995.

1996:

United Nations Children's Fund (UNICEF), *Plans of operation for health and nutrition services* HMG/N-UNICEF 1992-1996, New York, NY: UNICEF, 1996.

NOT DATED:

Agro-Forestry Basic Health and Co-operative (ABC/Nepal), *A Situation Analysis Report on "Girl Trafficking in Sindhupalchowk"*: Mahankal and Ichowk Village Development Committee, ABC/Nepal, Kathmandu, Nepal, n.d.

Agro-Forestry Basic Health and Co-operative (ABC/Nepal), *Red Light Traffic, The Trade in Nepali Girls*: ABC/Nepal, A Nepali

Women's NGO Working Against Girl Trafficking and AIDS, Kathmandu, Nepal, n.d.

T. Cox, *The Badi Prostitution as a Social Norm Among Untouchable Caste of West Nepal*, n.d.

K. Ellen, *Drums and Syringes, Shamans, Health Assistants and Patients in their Combat Against TB Bacilli and Hungry Ghosts in the Hills of Eastern Nepal*: Hovedfagsoppgave H-93, Socialanthropologisk Institute, Universitetsti Oslo, n.d.

P. L. Janssen, *The Role for NGOs in the Implementation of the National AIDS Programme in Nepal: A Study Into Factors Affecting Coordination*: National AIDS Programme in Nepal, Kathmandu, Nepal, n.d.

New Era, *A Study Report on Nepal Pharmacist Contraceptives Usage, Attitude and Distribution*: SOMARC, The Future Group, 1050 17th Street NW, Suite 1000 Washington, DC 20036, USA, n.d.

Save The Children (STC) (US), *Impact of the Save the Children (US) Non-formal Adult Education Programme on Mother and Child Health Care*: STC (US), Kathmandu, Nepal, n.d.

LIST OF NGOS SUPPORTED
BY AMFAR IN NEPAL
THROUGH 1995

Agro-forestry,
Basic Health and
Co-operatives (ABC/Nepal)
Kalikasthan
P.O. Box 5135
Kathmandu, Nepal
tel: 413934

Backward Society
Education (BASE)
Tulsipur, Rapti zone
Dang, Nepal
tel: 082-20055, -20043

B.P. Memorial Health
Foundation
(B.P. Memorial)
Pani Pokhari
P.O. Box 9694
Kathmandu, Nepal
tel: 415456

Center for Rural
Development and
Self Help (CRDS)
Siddhartha Nagar
P.O. Box 11
Nepal
tel: 071-21417

Child Development
Society (CDS)
Pipalbot Boudha
P.O. Box 2944
Kathmandu, Nepal
tel: 413460, 422644

Danuwar Sudhar Samiti
(DSS)
Pokhar Binda–1
Siraha, Sagarmatha
Lahan, Nepal
tel: C/O 047-20165 (Dudhauli)

Institute of Community
Health (ICH)
Tikapur
(Near Nepal Bank Limited)
Kailili, Nepal
tel: 091-60155 (request)

Lifesaving and Lifegiving
Society (LALS)
Dillibazar
P.O. Box 3517
Kathmandu, Nepal
tel: 413976

Nepal Center for Women and
Children Affairs (NCWCA)
Dhobhi Dhara
P.O. Box 15
Kathmandu, Nepal
tel: 416386

Nepal National Social Welfare
Association (NNSWA)
Kanchapur campus road
Ward no. 18
Mahakali zone, Nepal
tel: 099-22182, -21413

Nepal Society for Community
and Rural Development
(NESCORD)
Itahari, Nepal
tel: 025-80407

Sarwanam/Women's
Inspiration Community
(WICOM)
Gyaneshwor
P.O. Box 3955
Kathmandu, Nepal
tel: 410821

Social Awareness
for Education (SAFE)
Fultekra line, Ward no. 7
Nepalgunj, Nepal
tel: 081-21449

Women Acting Together
for Change (WATCH)
Old Baneswor
P.O. Box 5723
Kathmandu, Nepal
tel: 475653

Women's Rehabilitation
Center (WOREC)
Gaurighat
P.O. Box 4857
Kathmandu, Nepal
tel: 475815

Women's Self-Reliance
Center (MANK)
c/o Dipa Ranjani Rai
Action Aid Nepal
Lazimpat
P.O. Box 6257
Kathmandu, Nepal
tel: 011-61500 Public Call

LIST OF INTERNATIONAL NONGOVERNMENTAL ORGANIZATIONS AND INTERGOVERNMENTAL ORGANIZATIONS WORKING IN NEPAL

Action-Aid Nepal
Lazimpat
P. O. Box 6257
Kathmandu, Nepal
tel: 410929 fax: 419718

ADRA—Nepal
TNT Building, Top Floor
Teenkune
P. O. Box 4481
Kathmandu, Nepal
tel: 474380 fax: 410599

AIDSCAP—Nepal
Ram Shah Path
Putali Sadak
P. O. Box 8803
Kathmandu, Nepal
tel: 421371 fax: 421371

Asia Foundation Nepal
Baluwatar
P. O. Box 935
Kathmandu, Nepal
tel: 414813; 418345
fax: 415881

Asian Development Bank
Kamaladi
P. O. Box 5017
Kathmandu, Nepal
tel: 225063; 227779, -784

Canadian International
Development Agency (CIDA)
Lazimpat
P. O. Box 4574
Kathmandu, Nepal
tel: 415193, -389
fax: 410422

CARE—Nepal
Krishna Galli,
Pulchowk, Lalitpur
P. O. Box 1661
Kathmandu, Nepal
tel: 522143, -153;
523717, -718
fax: 521202

CECI—Nepal
Baluwatar
P. O. Box 2959
Kathmandu, Nepal
tel: 414430; 419412
fax: 413256

CEC/UoH —
STD/AIDS Project
Teku
P. O. Box 6331
Kathmandu, Nepal
tel: 232396; 233363

CEDPA—Nepal
Bhatbhateni
P. O. Box 5006
Kathmandu, Nepal
tel: 413156
fax: 421696

Danish Association
for International
Cooperation (DAIC)

Dillibazar
P. O. Box 4010
Kathmandu, Nepal
tel: 410040
fax: 411151

The Development Fund
P. O. Box 7647
Kathmandu, Nepal
tel: 419496
fax: 222976

Eastern Region PHC Project
Biz Bazaar, Dhankuta
Nepal
tel: 2620376

Friedrich Naumann
Foundation
Bhatbhateni
P. O. Box 3251
Kathmandu, Nepal
tel: 418610 fax: 419749

German Nepalese
Help Association
Thapathali Height
P. O. Box 3705
Kathmandu, Nepal
tel: 216908
fax: 226057

GTZ—Nepal
Pulchowk
P. O. Box 1457
Kathmandu, Nepal
tel: 523228-231
fax: 521982

HELVETAS—Nepal
Bakhundole Height, Kupon-
dole
P. O. Box 688
Kathmandu, Nepal
tel: 524925, -926
fax: 526719

John Hopkins University
J.H. U/P. C. S., Kalikasthan
P. O. Box 8048
Kathmandu, Nepal
tel: 414652
fax: 414652

Lutheran World Service
Kupondole Height,
Lalitpur
P. O. Box 3330
Kathmandu, Nepal
tel: 523861; 527212
fax: 523861

National AIDS
Prevention &
Control Project
Teku
tel: 215170; 226653
fax: 230406

OXFAM—Nepal
Sanepa Chowk
P. O. Box 2500
Kathmandu, Nepal
tel: 523197; 527230
fax: 527230

Plan International—Nepal
Doka Dal, Sanepa, Lalitpur
P. O. Box 1670
Kathmandu, Nepal
tel: 5216516; 535580
fax: 535560

Primary Health Care
Project Department
of Health Services
P. O. Box 1457
Teku, Pachali
Nepal

Private Agencies
Collaborating Together
(PACT)
Bhatbhateni
P. O. Box 5367
Kathmandu, Nepal
tel: 410473; 415244
fax: 410473

Redd Barna—Nepal
Ekantakuna, Jawalakhel
P. O. Box 3394
Patan, Nepal
tel: 521404; 524705
fax: 526359

Save the Children Japan
Baluwatar
P. O. Box 6935
Kathmandu, Nepal
tel: 421319; 422875
fax: 421319

Save the Children, U.K.
Chakupat, Patan
P. O. Box 992
Kathmandu, Nepal
tel: 521576, -591; 535159;
535161 fax: 527256

Save the Children U.S.A.
Maharajgunj
P. O. Box 2218
Kathmandu, Nepal
tel: 412447, -598; 415608
fax: 410375

SNV—Nepal
Kumaripati, Lagankhel
P. O. Box 1966
Kathmandu, Nepal
tel: 522915; 52344; 524597
fax: 523155

Social Welfare Council
Lainchaur
P. O. Box 2948
Kathmandu, Nepal
tel: 418111 fax: 410279

South Asia Partnership
Nepal
Old Baneshwor
P. O. Box 3827
Kathmandu, Nepal
tel: 476163, -671
fax: 471779

Swiss Development
Cooperation
Ekantakuna, Jawalakhel
P. O. Box 113
Kathmandu, Nepal
tel: 522020; 521428, –679;
524927-930; 526607
fax: 525358

Swiss Red Cross
Fateh Bal Eye Hospital,
Fultekra
P. O. Box 32
Nepalgunj, Nepal
tel: 081-20225

Unitarian Service
Committee of Canada
Baluwatar
P. O. Box 2223
Kathmandu, Nepal
tel: 414170
fax: 414170

United Mission to Nepal
Thapathali
P. O. Box 126
Kathmandu, Nepal
tel: 221379; 227016;
228060, -118
fax: 225559

United Nations
Development Program
(UNDP)
UNDP Building, Pulchowk
P. O. Box 107
Kathmandu, Nepal
tel: 523200

United Nations Fund
for Population Activities
(UNFPA)
UNDP Building, Pulchowk
P. O. Box 107
Kathmandu, Nepal
tel: 523637 fax: 523991

USAID
Rabi Bhawan
P. O. Box 5653
Kathmandu, Nepal
tel: 270144, -171; 271423,
- 425, -916; 272386
fax: 272357

World Bank
C/O Yak & Yeti Complex, Lal
Durbar
P. O. Box 798
Kathmandu, Nepal
tel: 222231; 223761;
226766, -792, -793
fax: 225112

World Education
Kamal Pokhari
P. O. Box 937
Kathmandu, Nepal
tel: 415790 fax: 415303

World Health Organization
UN Common Building
P. O. Box 108
Pulchwok, Lalitpur
tel: 523200/523993
fax: 523991